Reasons to Be an
OMNIVORE

For You and the Planet

Juan Pascual

"Man is the only creature
who refuses to be what he is."

Albert Camus
The Rebel

edra
PUBLISHING

Original title
Juan Pascual - Razones para ser OMNÍVOR. Por tu salud y la del planeta
© 2022 Grupo Asís Biomedia, S L
ISBN : 978-8-4191568-8-4

Book Publishing Manager: **Costanza Smeraldi**, Edra S.p.A.
Paper, Printing and Binding Manager: **Paolo Ficicchia**, Edra S.p.A
Cover: **Ursula Giusti**, Edra S.p.A.
Translation, Copyediting and Layout: **Star7 S.p.A**

©2024 Edra Publishing US LLC – All rights reserved
ISBN 978-1-962679-18-3
eISBN 978-1-962679-57-2

ed**ra**
PUBLISHING

Edra Publishing US LLC
3309 Northlake Boulevard, Suite 203
Palm Beach Gardens, FL, 33403
EIN: 844113980
info@edrapublishing.com
www.edrapublishing.com

Printed in Italy by Star7 S.p.A. Valle San Bartolomeo AL - Italia – August 2024

ABOUT THE AUTHOR

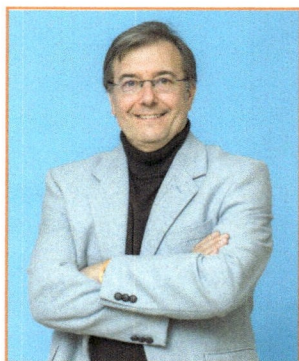

Juan Pascual (Barcelona, 1967) has a degree in veterinary medicine from the University of Zaragoza and an Executive MBA from IE Business School.

He started his career as a clinical veterinarian and later moved on to work in the animal health sector, where he has spent most of his professional life.

Within this field, he has worked in sales, marketing and management in several countries, including Italy, France and the United States as well as Spain and Latin America.

He has a significant presence on social media, where he comments on the key – yet often unknown – role played by animals in society and actively shares content on issues related to animal husbandry, animal welfare, pets and the importance of animal products in our diets.

He has published several articles on many science blogs, in cultural magazines and in many industry journals.

Juan is married and has four children.

For Charo

TABLE OF CONTENTS

FOREWORD

For 10,000 years, agriculture has been the backbone of civilization, providing the sustenance necessary for societies to flourish. Its impact extends far beyond the confines of fields and pastures, permeating the air we breathe and the biodiversity that sustains our planet. Within this vast and vital sector, livestock production holds a unique and influential position. Beyond the tangible nutritional benefits and environmental impacts, the cultural significance of livestock is profound. For many societies, animals represent more than mere sustenance; they are integral to cultural identity and heritage.

For most of human history, the goal of agriculture has been to produce more food to meet the needs of a growing and hungry population. Improvements in crop and livestock genetics, as well as new feeds and fertilizers, have dramatically increased yields and reduced hunger and poverty, but they have also come at a cost to the environment, health, and animal welfare. Addressing these global challenges while delivering safe, sufficient, appropriate, and nutritious food, requires new ways of producing food.

Fortunately, history shows that this is possible. Farming has changed dramatically over the last one hundred years in particular. The Green Revolution of the 1960s helped usher in many of these changes. While many people focus on the environmental consequences of the Green Revolution, it is worth considering what the world might have been like in the absence of such developments.

In 1970, Norman Borlaug, Father of the Green Revolution, won the Nobel Peace Prize for his contributions to saving a billion lives, but the environmental benefits of this revolution were also significant. For example, if the world were farming today with 1960s technology, we would need 1 billion additional hectares of land to feed the 8 billion humans on the planet, which would require cutting down as much as a quarter of all the forests on the planet. Innovation has allowed farmers to avoid such a disastrous outcome.

Through cooperation and collective effort, we can continue to devise solutions to the myriad issues confronting our planet. Effective communication is crucial in this endeavor—not merely talking, but engaging in meaningful dialogue that bridges divides and fosters genuine understanding. This book aims to facilitate such discussions, eschewing the sort of polarizing language that often hampers progress.

The disparities in meat consumption across the globe are striking and revealing of broader complexities within our food systems. In affluent regions where meat is abundant, reducing consumption may lead to significant environmental benefits and promote healthier lifestyles. Conversely, in areas grappling with nutritional deficiencies, increased access to animal-based foods can profoundly enhance health outcomes, helping to address critical issues such as stunting and cognitive impairment. In addition to the health and environmental issues at play, there are also economic and cultural factors that influence production and consumption. Livestock production is more than an agricultural activity; it is deeply embedded in the cultural fabric of many societies. These contrasting scenarios underscore the necessity for nuanced, region-specific solutions that reflect the complex realities of our global food systems.

The strength of our food system lies in its diversity—diversity of thought, approach, and practice. This diversity not only enriches our discussions, but also enhances our capacity to adapt and thrive in an ever-changing world. We must recognize that not all solutions will be universally accepted, nor do they need to be. Acknowledging that those with differing views are also striving to create a better future is a vital step toward mutual respect and understanding. It is sometimes sufficient to recognize our shared goals, even as we navigate diverse paths toward achieving them.

This book serves as a starting point for a more inclusive conversation about how we coexist with the animals that share our world and how we might continue to do so sustainably and ethically. It is a resource for those eager to engage in informed, thoughtful, and forward-thinking discussions about our place in the natural world and the myriad roles animals play in shaping the health and vitality of our societies. As we journey through these pages, let us seek understanding over confrontation, and unity over division, in our quest for a more balanced and sustainable coexistence.

Together, we can address the significant challenges before us. By reducing the environmental impact of meat production, while ensuring that nutritional needs are met globally, we can create a future where both people and the planet thrive. I hope you are inspired by this book, as I have been to join this vital conversation and contribute to a more sustainable and respectful dialogue about our food systems and our shared future.

Jack Bobo
Director Food Systems Institute University of Nottingham

FOREWORD TO
THE ORIGINAL EDITION

Humanity has had an intense relationship with animals, with whom it has shared territory and landscape, from the very beginnings of humankind.

First, as hunters and fishers throughout the Palaeolithic age, then, from the Neolithic period onwards, it was principally livestock farming that provided us with the meat, eggs and milk we needed. We took care of animals on livestock farms or we used animals like dogs and horses, to help us with various activities and functions. And that is how it was for thousands of years.

From the second half of the 20th century, accelerating at the start of the 21st century, a predominantly urban society removed from the countryside and livestock farming, started to "feel" a new relationship with animals. This resulted in the passing of successive laws, initially animal welfare laws and later animal rights laws, supported by an overwhelming majority in society. Initially, this seemed like a positive change. The issue, as always, is finding the balance between animal rights and the dietary and other needs of a growing global population.

This debate continues to rage. Readers of this book will enjoy a work that goes against the grain, questioning certain ideas that are accepted as incontrovertible truths about the use, position and contributions of domesticated animals in today's world. It takes a rigorous and detailed look at the relationship between humans and animals. Indeed, the role animals play in our society will undoubtedly take on a new dimension after you have read this book.

Today, although we share our homes with millions of pets, the urban world ignores animals' continued fundamental importance in society – the multiple industries that use their products, their importance in the development of medicines that save millions of lives, their role as pack animals in developing countries, and the contribution livestock make to the environment by consuming by-products or clearing the bush and scrubland.

The slaughter, which, until not long ago, was an occasion for celebration and involved a joint effort on the parts of families and neighbours, has disappeared from our lives or is presented to us in reports as something folkloric. We are unaware of the day-to-day reality of livestock farming, as if the steaks, sausages, eggs and milk appeared on the supermarket shelves every morning by magic. We undervalue farmers and their farms, while protesting if meat product prices increase in the supermarkets. Humanity has never been so far removed from the animals that fed it for millennia.

And it is this distance that causes us to have a distorted view of animals' – and indeed our own – position in society today. While the Renaissance put humans at the centre, making them the most important thing in the universe, today we are seeing a trend towards turning humans into just another animal. The separation between them and us is blurred and they, therefore, deserve to have to the same rights, to be treated the same. It is becoming increasingly common to hear animals referred to as "non-human people" in the media.

If we accept this paradigm, the conclusion is obvious: animals must be happy in the same way that we are, thus closing the circle that has led us from the anthropocentrism of the Renaissance to the anthropomorphism of today's animal rights movement, which puts animals on an equal footing with humans and rejects the idea of animals being owned or used for food or experiments. At the same time, the majority of people, unaware of this drift, receive these messages – which leave an impression – without seeing a counterpoint to them outside of specialist circles. This gives free rein then, for farmers to be portrayed as exploiters, scientists as torturers, and fishermen as murderers. Is that really the case? Do we rural people have to resignedly accept the demonisation of everything we do and represent?

That is why I recommend reading this book to listen to the voice of science and understand, in this light, our interactions with the animal world and the risk presented by prejudiced extremist attitudes that distort reality and show a profound lack of knowledge of animals.

Today's all-powerful and hubristic urban society cannot decide, with its simplistic ideals and fantasies, how farm animals should live. Some voices ask for the suppression of intensive livestock farming without considering the harm this would entail for the population's dietary needs.

We need to debate and argue the matter. Therefore, I highly recommend reading this book, which as I said at the start, goes against the grain but is revelatory due to the way it presents surprising information about the current status of animals and our society.

Dare to read it. It will certainly give you food for thought.

Manuel Pimentel Siles
Former Spanish Minister of Labour and Social Affairs

PREFACE

We all interact with animals on a daily basis, whether we are aware of it or not.

From the families that enjoy the company of their cat or dog, to all of us who consume products of animal origin (be it on our plates or in various products from a wide range of industries), to professionals involved in animal breeding and health and the scientists who need animals to develop medicines, we all bear witness to the key – yet often unknown – roles domesticated animals play in our society.

This human-animal interaction should be highly valued given that animals provide us with so many things, from companionship to vital nutrients, unique medicines and labour; indeed, tractors are still a rare sight today in many parts of the world. However, it is instead increasingly called into question by a part of society that sees in domesticated animals the main source of practically all the problems afflicting us: from climate change to cancer, hunger in many parts of the world and the loss of biodiversity. All these problems – and many other catastrophes – are linked to the consumption of animal products and animal breeding, and this vision is accepted as true – or at least viewed with sympathy – by a significant part of the population in the developed world. So much so that the animal rights movement is present in broad swathes of the political spectrum, since in Europe their principles are accepted by parties of all kinds, and its supporters have parliamentary representation in several countries.

Thinking about our relationship with animals is nothing new. The history of philosophy could perhaps be summarised as the attempt to find and explain what makes us human, different to them.

However, this is possibly the first time that the role animals play or should play in our lives is called into question and discussed in personal, societal and political spheres in the way it is today.

And, as a logical consequence, we see change by legislations paying a lot of attention to the animal world: farms, zoos, aquariums, pet shops, research laboratories, and even individuals' rights to own animals are all strictly regulated. But when we question animals' place in our world, we are also questioning humans' place in it.

Many of us have come across demonstrations or street stalls where animal rights activists show carefully selected photographs and videos showing what they describe as the "horrors" of animal experiments or animal husbandry to anyone who will pay attention to them.

Some textbooks, key instruments in the education of future generations, embrace these theories [1], making this vision "the reality" and the yardstick by which our students are graded.

And what is the response we, as citizens interested in animals, give to all these questions? How correct – or not – are these claims, some of which are accepted as absolute and verifiable truths as we have just seen? What arguments and data can we offer so that we can have a well-informed conversation and respond to these claims that are made so frequently, so visibly and so aprioristically?

What can we tell our children when they come back from school and tell us that their teachers have said that milk or meat production is bad for the planet and that cows or chickens or pigs are mistreated and live a life of terror?

The response we give – or don't give – to this question is likely to mould how future adults will see animals and their social role. If they don't receive any other message, they will grow up convinced that domesticated animals are an element we must dispense with if we want to build a better world.

The book you are holding doesn't just aim to be a book to read, it is intended to be a reference manual, and above all a manual for reflection, aimed at everyone interested in domesticated animals and their many contributions to our current society.

It is not so much about taking a position, instead it aims to introduce science into the conversation given that it has been largely removed from the debate, where ideology is now more important than a serene analysis of the data.

When we look at the animal world, we cannot forget the position, central or peripheral, we occupy in relation to it. Are we on the same moral plane? We are seeing ever more references in the media to studies that, theoretically, are progressively erasing the differences we thought existed between rational and irrational beings. According to these theories, human elements such as culture, language and consciousness are nothing more than characteristics that are more developed in *Homo sapiens* than in other species. They represent a difference in degree rather than a difference in nature between humans and the animal kingdom.

The driving idea behind this work is to provide the reader with a wealth of information, all based on scientific works published by leading international institutions or on studies by authors and publications of the highest prestige. This will give the reader a scientifically sound vision of the reality of domesticated animals in our society, of how much they contribute, of how their absence would inevitably lead to a much worse world, and of the differences not only of degree but also of nature that continue to exist between them and us. It is not necessary to convert animals into something they are not, or us into something we are not, in order to admire or love animals or to care or feel for them.

We all have the chance to influence, even if it is in a small way, how those around us think. If we do not respond with high quality information to messages that link animals to all the catastrophes afflicting the world, to messages that try to place them on the same moral plane as people (and consequently grant them equal rights), to the daily attacks that farmers, animal experiments, fishing and even those with pets are subjected to, then the media and public battle will be lost.

If the most radical theories prevail, animals will not live in better conditions, they will disappear. It is therefore vital to respond to these arguments that have become pervasive in society in general.

We all have a responsibility to provide a measured and reasoned response in our daily lives.

Society, and urban society in particular, which is largely ignorant of the reality of the animal world and its many contributions, will thank us, as will the animals that provide us with so much.

BY WAY OF INTRODUCTION

It was in October 2019 when, in a town hall meeting during the election campaign, US congresswoman Alexandria Ocasio-Cortez (AOC), who has been very active in the climate change mitigation movement, was interrupted by a militant who shouted at the audience: "We only have a few months left … to prevent global warming. We need to eat the babies…" AOC, visibly uncomfortable, couldn't hide her astonishment at a discourse that is not only not the best way to win votes – or donations – but also produces a deep, instinctive feeling of revulsion. While reducing human activity – including controlling birth rates – may be a potential option for reducing emissions, the mere mention of eating babies is, unquestionably, morally repugnant to the vast majority [2].

No less shocking is the proposal by the Swedish professor Magnus Söderlund that we should eat human cadavers to mitigate the effects of climate change [3].

These are only two examples – we could cite many more – of how the value of a human being is called into question by a part of the population that places humans at the same moral level, with the same value, as animals. Nevertheless, when all is said and done, the majority of us eat meat but not our fellow humans.

We can see that, if animals are on the same moral plane as people, then the logical conclusion is that their use, for example as food, will be called into question not only by animal rights activists but also by numerous media headlines. And the first step towards creating an anti-omnivore public opinion is making farming a scapegoat and promoting its limitation, or even its disappearance, as the solution to pollution, pandemics, fires in the Amazon, or unhealthy diets. Every solution to these problems involves getting rid of livestock, since it is responsible for all the ills afflicting humanity. Some even want to get rid of pets, as they too eat meat.

This book will provide the reader with a reference work for an educated and informed conversation about animal rights and its most common variant: veganism.

Some will find arguments they can use for an informed discussion with a relative who has embraced the cause. There are many parents who don't know how to respond when their child chooses to go vegan. With this book, they will be able to challenge the reasons behind such a decision.

However, beyond personal needs, this book aims to interrogate the content and consequences of this ideology because, while it is true that everyone should be free to choose what they eat or how they live, it's also true that the animal rights movement is managing to gradually impose some of its principles onto the real lives of thousands of people – especially children – without them having any chance to resist.

What some people present as positive and well-intentioned initiatives can lead to highly dubious results for the people who have to live with them, often without being consulted first. There are already numerous cities where school canteens limit meat consumption with the supposed aim of caring for the environment when what is really being neglected is the balanced, healthy and varied diet that schoolchildren deserve. Such initiatives include Meatless Monday, an initiative currently imposed in Baltimore, New York and Los Angeles [4], the attempt to impose vegetarian menus in state schools in the French cities of Grenoble and Lyon, and the imposition of vegan menus in a hospital in a British city [5].

We will look at the reasons why animals are given a moral status on a par with humans – especially in the most developed countries – and analyse the environmental, health and social consequences that the implementation of animal rights principles would – and indeed already do – have on society. We will also provide information and data so you can reflect in-depth and make informed arguments when involved in these conversations, which are becoming more and more common in the public and private spheres.

THE PLACE
OF ANIMALS
IN SOCIETY

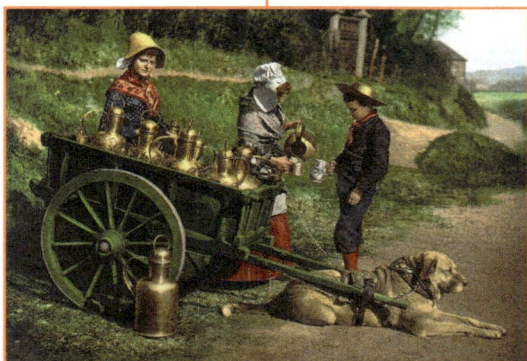

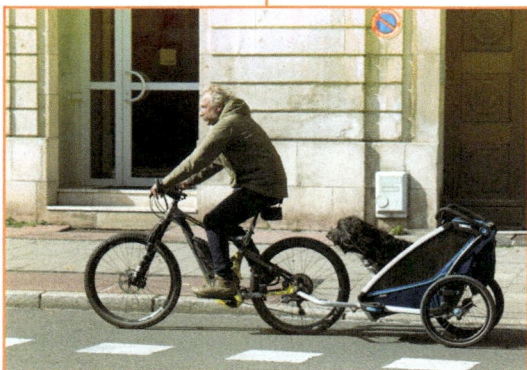

Change has been a constant throughout history. Societies evolve and what was routine at one time becomes a rarity years later. The societies of Ancient Egypt and Ancient Greece had a circular conception of time, and a lot of oriental cultures still do. However, in the West time moves in a straight line.

Other, less transcendental changes mould society. Until a few years ago, it was normal for aeroplanes and buses to have smoking and non-smoking sections. An absurd situation, but one we were all accustomed to at the time.

Technological progress in particular has a significant impact and is driving far-reaching transformations. Aviation, the contraceptive pill and, of course, the internet and social networks have resulted in incredible changes in how we interact with others and behave and relate to them.

If we consider the sacred to be what we would be prepared to kill or die for, we can say that, in the West, until fairly recently there were three things people were willing to make the ultimate sacrifice for: God, their Country and the Revolution. It's unlikely that there are many people who would give their lives for any of these ideas today in our geographical and cultural context.

It's possible that, these days, what we generally consider sacred and what a majority would be prepared to die for is our children. This wasn't the case not that long ago when children were part of the workforce and had no voice or vote within their families. In the USA, until the 1930s, insurance companies would compensate the death of a child with an amount calculated based on the value assigned to their work in the field [6].

On another note, until well into the 19th century, parents decided who their child would marry. Being free to choose who to marry and to do so for love didn't stop being an extravagance – that's how our ancestors would see it – until fairly recently [7].

What was normal a few decades ago now seems like an aberration.

We're now seeing another social change: our relationship with animals. Never before have they occupied such a key space in the lives of millions of people as they do today. The fact that we share our homes with cats and dogs hasn't just improved their lives – and the lives of a lot of people – it's also resulted in more attention and interest in domesticated animals in general. This attention and interest mainly comes from the urban world and leads to the projection of a distorted view of livestock farming in the rural environment. This distorted view has given rise to the animal rights movement as we know it today, which we will describe and analyse in more detail later.

We see the distance between the city and the countryside in the harshest light when we witness behaviours that are not just incomprehensible but profoundly contradictory in the rural environment; for example when inhabitants of big cities move to the country in search of peace and a slower pace of life then complain about a rooster crowing in the morning, as happened in France in 2017 [8]. The bird's owner won the court case and the incident led to the French parliament creating legislation that protects the sounds and smells of the countryside, such as the presence of dung, the noise of tractors or the crowing of the rooster Maurice, against the tide of urbanites ready to take to the courts. There have been more than 18,000 complaints of this nature in France alone in 10 years [9]. Such was the pressure that the mayor of a small town in the south of France put up a sign that read: "When we go to London we don't make Big Ben stop or stop Nôtre-Dame in Paris doing whatever it does. When you come to live in our small villages, you come to do just that and not to live in an aseptic world. We shouldn't forget that it is our farmers who grow the food we eat in France" [10].

> **The fact that we share our homes with cats and dogs hasn't just improved their lives – and the lives of a lot of people – it has also resulted in more attention and interest in domesticated animals.**

Spain has not escaped this trend either: a rural hotel complained about the owner of a chicken coop due to the sound of his poultry [11]. We can also see this trend in the lament of a sign put up by a Cantabrian farmer in her home town: "Churches have bells that work. Roosters are our rural alarm clock. Our animals cross streets and roads without notice. The cows wear bells that make noise. Farmers are working to guarantee that society has food to eat. Fertiliser smells bad when it is sprayed on the fields. Remember that you are in the countryside. Respect our customs, cultures and traditions [12]".

The perspective of the urban world has an ever increasing influence on the perception that most citizens have of animals.

The perspective of the urban world, which is after all where most of the population live and therefore where political power and the majority of voters are concentrated, has an ever increasing influence on the perception and conception that most citizens have of animals. So much so that it has become normalised in certain media to talk about non-human animals or even non-human persons. What are the consequences of this development, both from a moral (and, therefore, social) perspective and from a practical point of view? Is placing animals on the same moral, social and even legal level as humans always well-intentioned and innocent?

THE MORAL SUPERIORITY OF ANIMAL RIGHTS ACTIVISTS

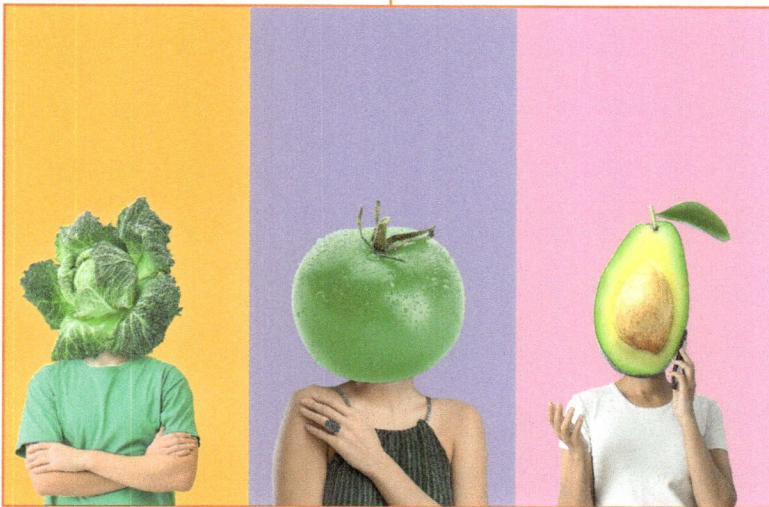

The vegan movement prides itself on being morally superior to those of us who eat an omnivorous diet. This book aims to challenge this claimed superiority which is shown to a greater or lesser extent by those who embrace the animal rights creed, and consequently follow a more or less strict vegetarian diet. In fact, the websites of their political parties and associations often allude to the morality of their actions and ideas. In 2018, for example, a joint statement by animal rights parties claimed:

> "… seventeen animal rights parties from across the world consider themselves morally obliged to publish a manifesto that alerts the whole planet of the terrible consequences of our current way of consumption [13]".

We can see a further example in the following extract from another animal rights organisation: "achieve ethical, social and legal guarantees, respect for animal integrity, welfare and rights [14]".

The academic world, which has numerous apostles of the vegan cause, is also responsible for similar comments. For example, Corine Pelluchon, a professor of philosophy at a Paris university, said in an interview: "The animal cause is at the heart of a new humanism [15]". Perhaps no other phrase sums up the profound sentiment behind this ideology better: anyone who does not integrate animal rights into their behavioural code is outside the boundaries of humanist thought.

Less academically, but with a greater media and visual impact, the US animal rights organisation PETA reflects the supposed ethical basis for its goals in its very name – the acronym stands for "People for the Ethical Treatment of Animals". Its website summarises what it means by the word ethical and does so with nothing less than a gospel source, specifically the Gospel of

Matthew 7:12 "Therefore whatever you desire for men to do to you, you shall also do unto them, for this is the law and the prophets". They also refer to the anti-racial segregation activist Martin Luther King Jr., using his phrase: "Injustice anywhere is a threat to justice everywhere". In this way, they imply that ethics must extend to mammals, reptiles, insects, crustaceans, molluscs, fish, birds and amphibians [16].

After all, a lot of vegans call themselves "ethical vegans" [17]. It is implicitly clear that it's difficult, if not impossible, for them to class anyone who doesn't share their culinary habits as ethical.

Since the cornerstone of the animal rights cause encourages the extension of the moral community – created by we humans – to include animals, those of us who do not embrace these ideas place ourselves outside the boundaries of ethical or moral behaviour (the two terms will be used synonymously in this book).

And we can therefore conclude that those who adopt this ideology see those of us who do not agree with their credo as alien to proper ethical behaviour and, therefore, morally inferior.

Such is the extent of radicalisation in some cases that the woman who led the 2015 Paris climate change summit, Costa Rican diplomat Christiana Figueres, declared: "How about restaurants in 10-15 years start treating carnivores the same way that smokers are treated? If they want to eat meat, they can do it outside the restaurant [18]. Crystal clear.

To finish with these examples, we'll take a look at the Dutch Party for the Animals, which has six seats in the national parliament. Their website explains their commitment to certain values, such as compassion [19]. Obviously, to disagree with their vision is to lack this virtue.

This party contributed to the creation and distribution of a documentary with the punning title *Meat the Truth* [20] [21] that repeats arguments about the impact of meat consumption on climate change that are full of inaccuracies and lack any scientific validity. They are preaching to the converted. I make this point because it's not a surprise that the cause's activists ignore objective data that reveals the claims, documentaries and advertisements they use to support their ideology to be false. PETA launched a campaign linking drinking milk with autism. This link was discredited by autism and nutrition experts [22]. We could fill an encyclopaedia with examples like the one above but, when it's a matter of defending a supposed ultimate good, distorting reality and twisting facts to advance the doctrine is permitted – the ends justify the means.

The media presence of animal rights activists permeates into society in such a way that some claims, although far from accurate, are perceived as being truths as solid as mathematical axioms.

At the end of the day, as Corine Pelluchon said at the vegan community's annual meeting in Paris [23], Veggie Pride 2017, "The scientific approach is not the only possible approach; you have to consider emotions too", (although later at the same event she appealed to ethology to demonstrate – scientifically this time – the similarities between humans and other animals) [24].

If objective data deserves the same consideration as subjective emotions, it's obviously unnecessary to appeal to the former to justify the latter.

However, the scientific evidence is stubborn and the information it provides us with is key, as it will enable us to evaluate the consequences of certain choices, for example, the majority embracing a diet without animal products.

We already know where these movements, parties and associations stand morally, ethically and humanistically. We will give a full response to the ideology they defend and demonstrate with data (we'll leave the emotions to the reader) that, contrary to what the majority may think, the consequences of a vegan diet and an animal rights-based approach to society would have – does have – profoundly negative consequences both for people and, above all, for the animals they want to defend. What's more, it does not achieve a positive counterbalance either for the health of the people who adopt these diets or for the health of the planet.

It's not easy to make yourself heard given the media presence of animal rights activists and the attention that the vegan movement gets in the media. This then permeates into society in such a way that some claims, although far from accurate, are perceived as being truths as solid as mathematical axioms.

In January 2003, I went to the International Poultry Exposition for professional reasons. This is an annual poultry convention attended by veterinarians, breeders and, in short, the entire poultry producing industry. In the morning, close to the hall where the events were being held, a small group of people protested against the abuse that they believe the poultry industry inflicts on birds. There were no more than a dozen people, some dressed as chickens, and they were carrying a few signs. Yet, in the evening, the protesters were mentioned in all the local news programmes.

This example shows that media attention can enable the message to gradually permeate into society that every animal on every farm is always suffering or that the consumption of meat is, like one of the ten plagues of Egypt, harmful for our health and the environment.

BEING VEGAN: A DIFFICULT CHOICE

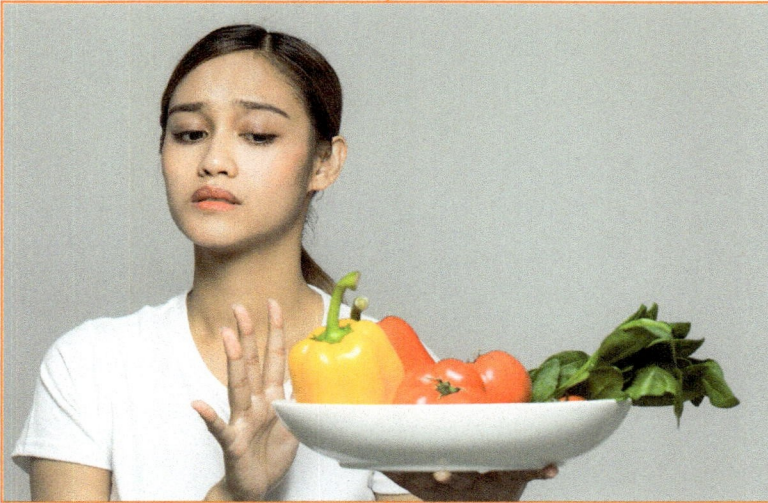

Perhaps this tendency to place themselves on a higher moral plane is born of the need to compensate for the numerous sacrifices the vegan cause demands. After all, throughout our whole evolution humans have eaten huge quantities of meat when we've had the opportunity. Meat was so important that the earliest cave paintings show hunting scenes and the animals being hunted. In fact, palaeontologists today agree that eating meat is what made us human beings [25] [26]. That's because the nutritional richness and energy density of meat allowed us to reduce the size of our intestine and, at the same time, increase the size of our brain. So, it was the carnivorous diet that made *Homo sapiens* develop into what they are today.

So it's not surprising that it's hard to give up foods of animal origin. In fact, 84% of people who try vegetarianism (or the vegetarian lifestyle as some prefer to call it) give it up [27] [28]. The reasons behind this are varied: from difficulties implementing their diet to deterioration in their health, which is the most frequently cited reason [29].

A not insignificant number say they decided to give up veganism because they feel the need to eat animal products as they admit they didn't feel well or feel satiated by meals lacking animal products. Here are two accounts by way of example:

"I was always hungry no matter how large my bowl of beans and rice. Even worse than constant hunger, I didn't seem to enjoy food the way other people did. Eating was a chore, like folding laundry or paying bills, but even more annoying because if I didn't do it I would die. I was sick of being hungry, I was sick of beans and rice, and so at the age of 31, I have made a decision: I will try and become a meat eater. [28]"

The author Lierre Keith, who followed a vegan diet for 20 years, said: "(a vegan diet) is not sufficient nutrition for long-term maintenance and repair of the human body. To put it bluntly, it will damage you. I know. Two years into my veganhood, my health failed, and it failed catastrophically [30]".

Evidently, this is not an experience shared by all vegans but we can say that the majority give up veganism and, furthermore, that they do so within a few months of starting their new lifestyle [31]. A lot of them claim to have felt seriously unwell following this diet and others, enthusiastic influencers who support the diet, are caught eating animal products. This was the case with the well-known instagrammer Rawvana who, with more than two million followers on her YouTube and Instagram accounts, admitted to having incorporated fish and eggs into her diet for medical reasons [32].

84% of people who try the vegetarian diet (or the vegetarian lifestyle as some prefer to call it) give it up.

No less curious, due to the duplicity it demonstrates, is the case of the New York restaurant Eleven Madison Park, whose chef decided to remove animal products from its menu because in his own words: "The current food system is not sustainable". However striking such a statement from the capital of tarmac may seem, it's even more surprising that a local journalist discovered that this very same establishment offered a menu with meat, shellfish and all kinds of delicacies in a private dining room reserved for millionaire customers [33].

Staying in the USA, in 2014 ex-president Bill Clinton abandoned the vegan diet he had adopted in 2011 following the advice of his doctors – it's curious how doctors advise giving up a vegan diet but never an diet. This did not prevent prominent leaders of vegan associations from declaring that they continue to count him as a member of these associations since, after all, "We applaud everyone doing the best they can" [34], even though this permissiveness is not usually shown to ordinary mortals.

The results on this side of the Atlantic are not that different. A survey [35] published in France in May 2021 by an organisation reporting to the French Ministry of Agriculture with more than 15,000 respondents from France reported that 2.2% of the total population are vegetarians, and vegans represent a minute minority of this number, making up 0.3% of all the people surveyed. It's revealing to see how, according to this survey, 45% of vegans admit that they break the rules of the diet now and again and eat products of animal origin.

Studies indicate that in the USA, 2% of the population are vegans and 2% vegetarians [36], figures that are very similar to the European numbers.

There's no doubt that the vast majority of us like meat, milk and eggs and that the people who give them up buy substitutes that imitate them. By their own admission, they also suffer a deterioration in their health in many cases and have to take vitamin supplements (especially B vitamins) to replace vitamins only found naturally in products of animal origin.

We often see headlines in the media announcing the explosion of the vegetarian diet, for example in 2018, *The Independent* reported that millions of Britons were now vegans [37]. Nevertheless, meat consumption data from the UK show how actual behaviour differs significantly from what respondents say in surveys – meat consumption in the United Kingdom has not stopped increasing since the year 2000 [38].

Giving up flavoursome foods and replacing them just with vegetables is a big challenge, as shown by the fact that vegans often have dreams related to the consumption of meat [39]. Having to take vitamins and minerals routinely is also difficult, as is having to subject yourself to regular tests to check whether there has been a decrease in these vital nutrients in your body.

The reality is that there aren't many vegans and that a large majority who try veganism give it up. Nevertheless, their media presence – and therefore their political influence – is very significant given their meagre numbers.

BEYOND
ALTRUISM

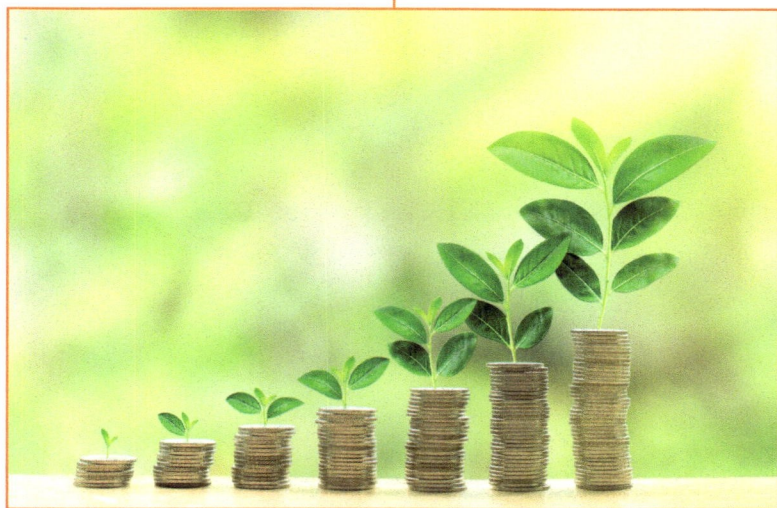

It's noteworthy how vocal this minority is. They have undoubtedly gained a great deal of public attention with very visual and eye-catching actions and demonstrations that have been a magnet for the media, who in turn have become, willingly or not, loudspeakers for this cause. Militants locking themselves in cages or trying to simulate a slaughterhouse with red paint and ketchup, demonstrations showing dead piglets or "goodbyes" organised at the gates of slaughterhouses are frequent events that see their limited success in terms of attendance multiplied by their disproportionate presence in the media.

But it's not all altruism. In fact some organisations from this school of thought, such as Open Philanthropy launched by Dustin Moskovitz – one of the co-founders of Facebook and a militant vegan – give donations amounting to millions of dollars to certain media, such as The Guardian or the *Nine Media Group*, so that they produce slanted articles and videos showing negative aspects of livestock farming [40] [41].

The Silicon Valley Community Foundation, which receives millions of dollars of donations from the CEOs of companies such as Facebook and GoPro, send funds to several European animal rights organisations, up to $12.8 million in 2017 alone [42].

In France, the total budget of animal rights associations is €21 million. If we add the amounts managed by organisations for the protection of animals and the environment, the total figure rises to almost €100 million.

And it's not as if there's only altruistic interests at play in animal rights activism. We also have the example of the NGO Vegan Action, which is responsible for certifying products to guarantee to consumers that they do not contain products of animal origin. Their revenue in 2018 was $1.3 million [43].

VEGANISM
AS A RELIGION

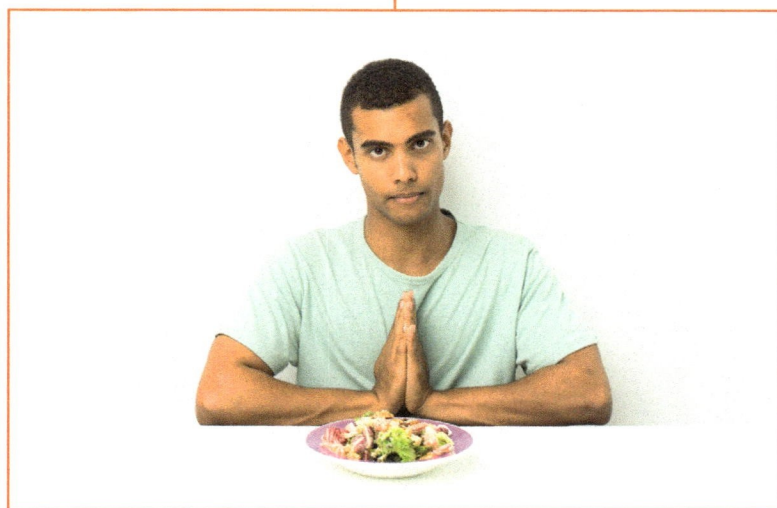

Given their proselytising nature and the higher moral plane that they place themselves on (certainly their associations do, as we have seen), it's not surprising that the behaviour of a lot of vegan groups (including political parties) borders on the religious.

At least two judges - one in the UK and one in the US state of Ohio - have ruled that giving veganism the same legal protection as religion is legitimate: both cases, albeit for different reasons, the defendants refused to follow the corporate guidelines of the companies that employed them, citing their vegan ideology.

In the case in England the trigger was a disagreement about investments that his company's pension fund had made in companies that conduct animal testing. In the case in Ohio, an employee of a hospital refused to get a flu shot, claiming that embryonic eggs were used to replicate the virus needed to produce the vaccine.

Judges consider that, although being a vegan did not entail belief in a superior being or worship, the practice could be recognised and have the same rights as religious beliefs

In both cases, the judges ruled that, although being a vegan did not entail belief in a superior being or worship, the practice could be recognised and have the same rights as religious beliefs. In other words, vegans have the right not to be discriminated against because of their beliefs since, for their followers, these beliefs determine what is good and what is bad, much like religious beliefs,.

These rulings open up previously unknown possibilities. For example, with these precedents, an employee of a supermarket could refuse to handle any packaging containing products of animal origin. That wouldn't just affect the food section, it would also affect the beauty, clothing and medicine sections. In other words, it would affect practically every section given that numerous animal substances are used in countless industrial processes, as we shall see later on.

It is also striking that animal rights activists are scandalised by the supposed mistreatment some animals might be subjected to while staying silent about other products that are ethically more reprehensible, simply because they affect human welfare. There are a lot of unjust situations in the world, and a lot of products that are the result of abuse. In fact, the origin of the batteries in the mobile phones we all have in our pockets has been criticised by Amnesty International [46], but for animal rights activists only the defence of animals seems worthy of their time. Even then there are exceptions, seeing as they continue to consume avocados even when their cultivation, in some cases, affects the free movement of elephants [47]. Nor do they stop consuming coconut milk even though some coconuts are harvested by systematically mistreated monkeys [48].

Most religions make an effort to gain followers. Some of them even make proselytising an essential practice because attracting new believers is a duty. This drive to gain new followers is also common among vegans. There are countless associations that invite us to join their cause and, in Europe in particular, there are several political parties that include vegetarianism and animal rights in their political ideology.

History is full of examples in which different creeds have persecuted people of different faiths: Catholics and Huguenots in 16th century France, the expulsion of Jews from England in the 14th century, or from Spain and Portugal in the 15th century. Even today, some strands of Islam call for the elimination of infidels.

Today, however, for most faiths, anyone who shares them is a brother and anyone who doesn't is someone worthy of commiseration, since they are missing out on the benefits that religion promises. Nevertheless, they still must be loved and listened to because they are inherently precious and deserve to be urged to join the cause.

NOT ALWAYS
A KIND FACE

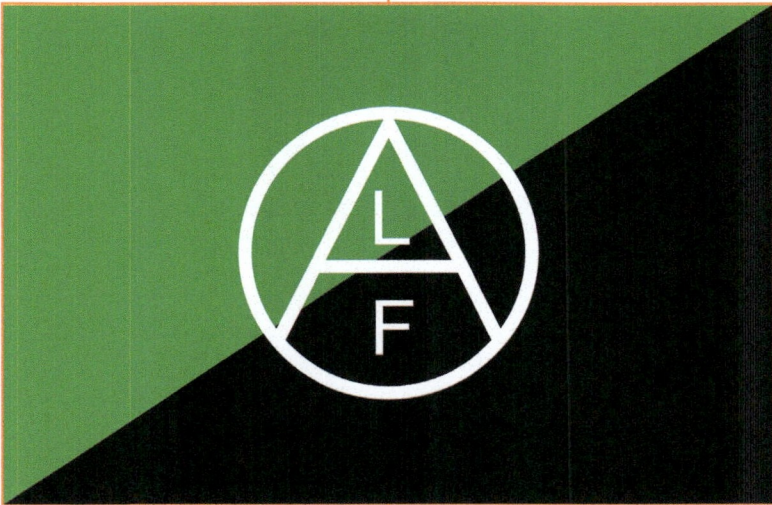

But animal rights activism in general is inflexible with anyone who doesn't share its principles. You're either with them or you are against them. The level of aggressiveness shown by some activists on social networks, in their own advertising campaigns, and in statements to the press is shocking. Anyone who thinks there should be a difference in the moral treatment of humans and animals is called a speciesist (putting them on the same scale as racists and sexists). People who use animals for experiments are called torturers and those who work in zoos or aquariums are described as prison guards [49] [50] [51]. We could also add the absolute lack of respect some of these militants have shown after the death of bullfighters [52].

And we shouldn't forget the harassment former vegans, such as the Canadian gymnast and blogger Maddie Lymburner and the British athlete Tim Shieff, have been subjected to. They suffered all manner of attacks and insults on social networks when they announced that they were incorporating animal products into their diet. Anyone who renounces, like apostates, is condemned to the most radical ostracism [53]; all very fraternal, empathic and humanist.

In contrast, other groups that defend causes considered noble and morally unquestionable by a large majority, such as the abolition of the death penalty, act very differently: they try to convince people who do not share their views, but they don't insult or act aggressively towards those they disagree with.

After all, we shouldn't forget that animal rights groups have flirted with terrorism. The most illustrative case is the Animal Liberation Front (ALF), an animal rights organisation considered by US and UK authorities to be a terrorist organisation. Without going to the extreme of directly targeting people, it has participated in numerous acts of sabotage and has even been responsible for bombings. Its manuals, which can be downloaded from its website, focus in particular on the fur industry and explain in detail where farms and their suppliers are located, with names and telephone numbers of employees and clear instructions on how to do as much damage as possible in order to drive them to ruin [54].

In 2005, one of their magazines, *Bite Back*, published a direct action report stating that in 2004 alone FLA activists had "liberated" 17,262 animals and carried out 554 acts of vandalism and arson [55]. This website continues to be active and describes each "direct action" they carry out in detail: ranging from "liberating" animals, covering shop windows in red paint and hacking IT systems of "enemy" companies, to attacking butchers' shops and puncturing the tyres of hunters' cars [56].

The constant attacks by the animal rights world against the livestock sector – calling farmers exploiters, cruel and torturers – have contributed to agriculture's loss of prestige and have found a powerful platform in the media

These violent actions find support in some academic circles. Although the majority of philosophers who embrace vegan positions are pacifists, others call pacifism obsolete. Steven Best, professor of humanities and philosophy at the University of Texas claims that militant direct action is a form of self-defence and gives the example of soldiers from some African countries who deter poachers by using weapons and, in this way, protect species at risk of extinction, such as elephants and rhinoceroses [57]. From this perspective, he shamelessly claims that the slogan "violence only creates more violence" is a pacifist myth. Best's extreme positions (one of his books was titled *Terrorists or Freedom Fighters? Reflections on the Liberation of Animals*) were enough to make him *persona non grata* in the United Kingdom.

The constant attacks by the animal rights world against the livestock sector – calling farmers exploiters, cruel and torturers – have contributed to agriculture's loss of prestige and, as we have seen, have found a powerful platform in the media. It's not an innocent movement, the consequences can be counted in human lives. For example, in France more than 600 farmers commit suicide every year [58] [59]. Of course, the causes are many and varied, among them the economic difficulties of the sector, but the impact of the loss of social prestige associated with a job that is absolutely essential to society and yet is seen by many as harmful to the environment and to livestock is not insignificant on this ultimate, drastic decision.

DOMESTICATED ANIMALS AND HUMANS: A SYMBIOTIC RELATIONSHIP

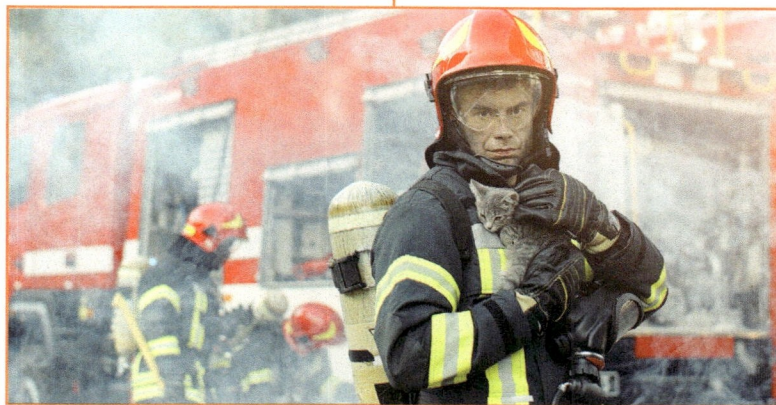

However, beyond the free choice as to what we decide to eat or not - which everyone has the right to and which we should all respect is it true that being a vegetarian is morally better than being an omnivore? I am going to answer this question from two different perspectives.

Firstly, I will look at the debate regarding animal rights. Are animals in the same moral category as humans? Is using animals the way we do correct from a moral perspective?

Secondly, I will describe what a world without domesticated animals would look like. Would it be a better world? What would the consequences of dispensing with their services be, for example for food, testing, and transport? Ultimately, the answer we get should guide our behaviour.

There is no doubt that animals deserve respect. Harming them without a good reason is reprehensible, a crime recognised in a lot of countries. It's only right that this is the case.

Therefore, special attention should be paid to the animals that live among us, either in farms or in our homes, because as domesticated animals they depend on us, and their welfare is our responsibility.

Some philosophers argue that we should also be worried about the welfare of wild animals and that predation is inherently negative given that an animal suffers when it is attacked by another animal and, therefore, we should eradicate the possibility of this. They suggest that predators should be sterilised [60] or that we should gradually change the behaviour of some predators, for example some birds could be taught to eat soya worms so that they do not feed on earthworms [61]. The catastrophic ecological consequences these initiatives could have don't seem to merit the attention of the pseudointellectuals who propose them.

Despite some more or less extravagant suggestions, there is no doubt that wildlife and the ecological mechanisms it involves can be, to our eyes, cruel and violent.

Before we look at the moral value of animals, it is vital that we understand the different interactions they have with us, both in the countryside and in the city. Examining these interactions will provide us with a basis for understanding whether or not – or to what extent – they are morally reprehensible and whether their presence in coops, pastures or apartments makes the world a better or worse place.

THE BRUTALITY OF THE WILD

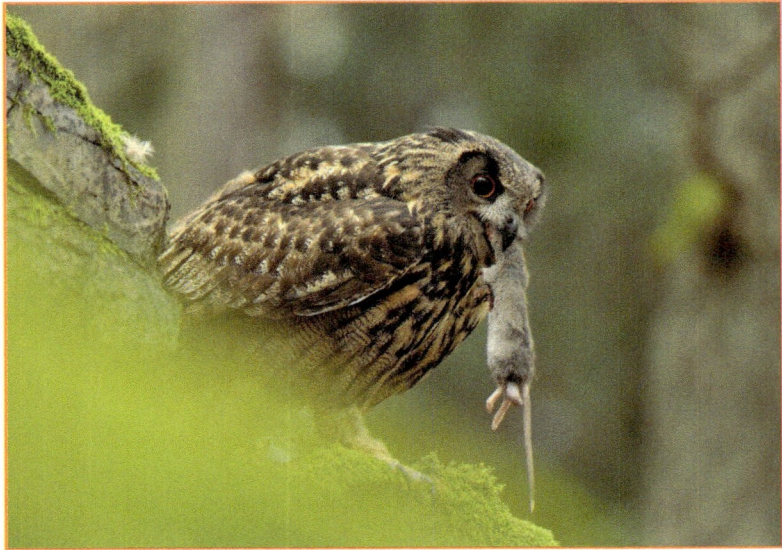

Let's travel for a moment to the beaches of Namibia. The southern spring sees the arrival of a new generation of seals. The pups have just been born and the mothers are faced with two urgent challenges: providing food for their young while, at the same time, protecting them by being with them as much as possible because they are surrounded by predators waiting to snatch them away at the slightest slip. Jackals and hyenas are on the prowl. But there's another threat, much less obvious but no less dangerous for the seal pups: seagulls. The birds circle over the young pups with one goal: to eat the pups' eyeballs. A seagull can't eat a seal pup but it won't hesitate to perch on it in order to pluck out, with two quick and precise pecks, the bundle of proteins and fluids that make up the pup's eyeballs. The pup, blinded, is now easy prey for any other predators that join the feast and sink their jaws into its defenceless body. A scavenger will eat its remains, but even if doesn't fall prey to these predators it will die of infection or starvation because its mother will refuse to feed it because it has no chance of survival. And resources are scarce for seals [62].

Animals deserve respect. Harming them without a good reason is reprehensible, a crime recognised in a lot of countries. It's only right that this is the case

Let's go now to Yellowstone National Park in the USA. Here a wolf pack is exhausting a bison's stamina. They've been stalking it for hours and the bison is at its limit. The wolves bite the bison's legs to immobilise it and start to eat it alive. It's not easy for a wolf to give a fatal bite and kill such a beast, so the battle drags out over hours of adrenaline and hours of fierce fighting for survival. The enormous bison has little chance of escape and even if it does, it will die as a result of the numerous bites it has received. The bison suffers a slow death until sepsis invades its tissues, and it succumbs to infection [63].

But the wild is savage for predators as well. If the wolves don't succeed, their pups will die of starvation. Seventy percent of wolf pups die before reaching 12 months of age [64].

Fate is no easier on a lion hit in its jaw by an accurate zebra kick. The toothless feline will die of hunger and thirst and may even meet its end trampled by a buffalo herd or devoured by hyenas [65].

However, we don't have to go far to find examples of how nature can be absolutely ruthless. In our gardens, praying mantises hold other insects – and even their own mate – in their powerful forelegs and eat them alive. A chick falls from its nest and is rapidly covered and dismembered by ants.

It's wrong to think that predators kill their victims to be "humane"; they do it because it's safer to eat a dead zebra than a live one. Dead prey won't try to kick or gore the predator and potentially break one of their bones. There are several examples that show animals eating their prey live if they don't represent a risk to their physical integrity [66] [67].

No, nature is not kind. Human beings have spent millennia trying to tame it so they don't fall victim to it. The philosophers of the Age of Enlightenment had it crystal clear. Nature was seen as hostile: droughts, pestilence, earthquakes, plagues. All these natural elements put human life at risk [68]. In the words of Voltaire after the earthquake that laid waste to Lisbon in 1755: "Man must tame nature to be master of his own destiny".

Today, to a large extent, we have done so: we live longer and better, we have cures for a lot of diseases and wild animals are not as common a danger as they were in earlier times. However, the wilderness is still there, and those who live in it have to fight for every morsel, for every breath in a life-or-death battle to raise their offspring, to survive another day and to increase their odds of passing on their genes to the next generation.

I have described a few cases – in reality there are innumerable such cases – to demonstrate that life in the wild for animals is far from a happy Arcadia [69]. The most common cause of death for herbivores is being eaten by a predator. A predator, when it can't hunt, will die of hunger. In either case, disease may hit at any moment and strike them down. Millions of young die because their mothers can't feed them or fall victim to a predator. And that's how life in the wild works, there's nothing to complain about.

The most common cause of death for herbivores is being eaten by a predator. The only option for a predator when it can't hunt is to die of hunger

Contrast the life of farm animals and, of course, pets with these scenarios. They are not a homogeneous group, as the animals' circumstances vary greatly depending on their function, owners and location. For example, the circumstances of a sow living and farrowing in a windowless pigsty in the backyard of a farmhouse in China, the ox resting after a long day pulling the plough in Pakistan and the chicken fattened on a modern farm in the US state of Arkansas are very different. However, they all have something in common: someone else worries about providing them with food. They have intrinsic value, either because they produce milk, meat, eggs, honey or wool etc. or because we use their strength to work the fields, carry heavy loads and as a means of transport. After millennia of selection, the majority of domesticated animals (the few species that can be domesticated) could not return to life in the wild. They would simply perish; they would not know how to feed themselves and they would not know how to escape from predators. We could say the same of some domesticated animals we keep as pets, for example some breeds of dog. To take a more extreme example, silkworms, domesticated in China some 9,000 years ago, are no longer found in the wild. Only the domestic varieties exist [70].

DOMESTICATION: A SYNERGISTIC PROCESS

It may be arguable whether the life of domesticated animals is worth living, but there's no doubt that it is less stressful and tough than the lives of the majority of their wild counterparts.

We could say that these animals trust us to give them food in return for their products or brute strength. We both benefit. As well as food, domesticated animals also receive protection against predators (it couldn't be any other way since the predators are competing directly against humans, which has led us on many occasions to fight them with real ferocity). The domesticated animal is also protected against bad weather since modern farms have heating and cooling systems, and they also get veterinary care – especially in more developed countries.

In exchange for what we might define as benefits, domesticated animals in some cases, have some limitations to their freedom to move, they cannot reproduce as their biology dictates, they will be with their offspring for a limited time, and their life expectancy will be determined by when they have to leave their farm and head for the slaughterhouse.

Domestication has been a synergistic process. The fact is that the species that have been able to domesticate have had resounding evolutionary success – their numbers have increased exponentially proving this. To give one example, while it has been estimated that there are approximately 400,000 wolves in the world, there are an estimated 800 million of their evolutionary cousins, dogs [71].

The animals we have been able to domesticate had some predisposition to it. For example, a wild horse will allow a human to approach it until they are as little as 17 metres away, while a zebra flees when a person is still 37 metres away [71]. As the domestication process progresses, the selection of genes linked to docility – we select animals we can control – is associated with the development of other physical characteristics, which Darwin described as domestication syndrome [72], namely: animals with floppy ears, flattened snouts or the appearance of white patches in their coat. More recently, we have discovered that, since they don't have to worry about predators, domesticated animals have a smaller brain – with no predators lurking they can afford to. They also secrete less testosterone – a sign of suffering less stress than their wild counterparts [71].

> Domestication has been a synergistic process. The fact that the species that it has been possible to domesticate have had resounding evolutionary success – their numbers have increased exponentially – is proof of this

There is no doubt that the domestication of dogs started when these animals started to approach human settlements. In other words, the animals themselves contributed to their own domestication: to a certain extent (and to varying degrees depending on the species) they looked for coexistence with humans and proximity to them.

Millions of domesticated animals live in extensive farms: they could escape and live in the wild (we have examples, such as some horses in the USA) but the vast majority stay in their flocks or herds because they know food and protection against predators is guaranteed if they live alongside humans.

Some may find this undesirable, as they advocate the abolition of all forms of animal husbandry and of all forms of animal ownership. However, it's indisputable that livestock farming and the animals that live with us in our cities give billions of animals the chance to live. The alternative would be for these billions of animals to disappear.

It's a curious way for animal rights activists to defend animals: advocating for their disappearance.

However, if this did happen and livestock animals disappeared – as some fervently want – they would be replaced in many regions by wild animals. When extensively farmed livestock is not present, its space is occupied by wild ungulates. These wild animals would live as such: at the mercy of predators and diseases, and without the protection animals raised by humans enjoy. So, if livestock are eliminated, their wild substitutes would have a lower quality of life, which for some would be questionable from a moral perspective.

We have seen that wild animals have a much worse life than domesticated animals but how do animals live in a farm beyond having food and shelter? How high is their quality of life? Aren't farms a breeding ground for infections for animals and a risk for humans as well? Do we really have a symbiotic relationship with animals, or do we abuse them?

CONSEQUENCES OF LIVESTOCK FARMING FOR ANIMALS

The reality is that a large majority of livestock farmers live with their animals, work with and for them 365 days a year, and go out of their way to care for them. In a lot of cases without holidays or weekends.

The vast majority do it to wrest something of value from the soil. There are billions of people on earth who get their proteins, vitamins, minerals and all kind of high-value nutrients thanks to livestock farming. There are people who don't have access to supplements or vegetables that contain these nutrients and who, without animals, would simply be malnourished.

Let's analyse an aspect that animal rights activists – or the vast majority of them – claim is an indisputable truth, an obvious reality:

"Every farm animal suffers, on every farm in the world. Always. Therefore, we have to eliminate animal production".

This principle abounds in every work by animal rights philosophers. For them it is an axiom that, like in the mathematical world, is a self-evident truth and, therefore, does not need to be proven.

Well, we're going to remove the cornerstone of this building. And, as we'll see, without it, the whole edifice comes crashing down.

Animal rights activists' axiom that all farm animals are always suffering is, purely and simply, an unsubstantiated fallacy, as anyone who has a minimum amount of experience with animals will know

Anyone that has ever visited a farm will know that it's absurd to claim that all animals in farms are always suffering. When we see sheep grazing in the fields in summer or cows in the meadow, we're not looking at frightened animals nor even evasive creatures trying to escape their environment. In fact, cows return to the milking parlour by their own volition when it's time to do so and, if the farm has a robotic milker, they even milk themselves when they want to. There's no doubt that some animals can be stressed, or in pain or discomfort. An infection, a sprain or the midday heat in the south or the cold of the mountain are not pleasant. But that doesn't mean their life is hell and isn't worth living.

There are a lot more cases, and we'll look at some later on. Nevertheless, what we can confirm is that animal rights activists' axiom that all farm animals are always suffering is, purely and simply, an unsubstantiated fallacy, as anyone who has a minimum amount of experience with animals will know.

Since the animal rights world claims that the absence of welfare is the norm and its supporting philosophy is based on this idea, let's take a closer look to see whether it's really true and try to understand the ethical aspects linked to the welfare of domesticated animals.

ANIMAL WELFARE

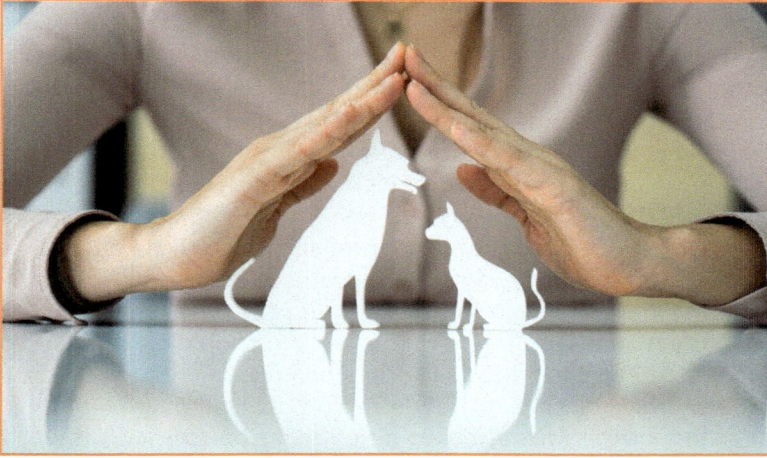

Animals are beings capable of feeling fear, pain, hunger, etc. and we have the moral obligation to prevent them feeling these sensations as far as possible. In more developed countries, both legislation and the operating procedures of the production companies themselves aim to do this. It is right that this is the case. Domesticated animals are our responsibility, they depend on us and, therefore, it's not enough that they have a better life than they would in the wild (which as we have seen can be truly horrifying). Instead, we must treat them with respect and try to provide them with the best possible care and living conditions, whilst maintaining the economic viability of the farm – otherwise their chances of subsistence will simply vanish.

The preoccupation with farm animals' quality of life was passed into law when the British government introduced, in 1965, what it called the *five freedoms* that all domesticated farm animals must be guaranteed. These freedoms are:

• Freedom from hunger and thirst
• Freedom from fear and distress
• Freedom from physical or thermal discomfort
• Freedom from pain, injury or disease
• Freedom to express normal behaviour

61

We could debate *ad nauseam* whether these freedoms are respected on farms or not. However, it is unquestionable that animals get closer to these freedoms on farms than they do in the wild.

A wild bird or antelope is rarely free of fear. It will live in a constant state of alert to avoid being heard, seen or smelled by a predator. On the other hand, predators spend most of their life with an acute feeling of hunger that compels them to hunt and risk their life from a goring or kick to their eye or their jaw from their prey. Needless to say, the discomfort of the seasons takes its toll on their quality of life. Certainly, they will be able to express their normal behavioural patterns but let's not forget that these behaviours include fleeing from predators, and it doesn't seem reasonable to argue that a chicken should be exposed to a fox so that it can "express normal behaviour". So, the five freedoms have their caveats but there's no doubt that the legislation and the industry itself makes an effort to comply with them, at least in our part of the world. It's also the case that an animal with a high level of welfare will perform better and ultimately be more profitable for the people who bred it.

So, for example, in the European Union (EU), the legislation does not permit piglets to be weaned at less than 28 days of age, which is a right a newborn child does not have [73].

Or the law being prepared in Germany for approval in 2024, which will prohibit chick sexing from the seventh day of incubation as there is evidence that the embryos feel pain from this time [74]. Remember that abortion is legal in Netherlands until the 24th week – and beyond in some cases. I'm not trying to make a comparison between the legal treatment of human and chick embryos. The reader can draw their own conclusions.

The concept of the five freedoms is being questioned by specialists. For example, hunger is seen as a negative condition from this perspective. However, the feeling of hunger is vital for triggering the impulse to eat and is only a problem if it's prolonged and a potential cause of suffering. As a result, five domains of animal welfare have been proposed. This model makes emotions the key factor in animal welfare [75].

Defining animal welfare is not an easy task. It's not even easy to define human welfare. We can be physically healthy but sad because our football team has lost or because we're in pain from surgery, or be happy because our child has graduated from university. There's no doubt that welfare is based on objective and subjective sensations. This means it's relatively easy to conclude whether an animal is in good physical condition but rather more difficult to know if they are comfortable, stressed or in fear.

At this point, it's vital to stress that the aim is to determine what the animal prefers and not what we think its preferences would be. This point is critical because it must be the animal that shows us what it prefers. Let's look at two examples:

There are two laying hen production systems in Europe. Firstly, we have enriched cage production: these cages allow the animal to extend their wings and have litter for the hen to scratch and a nest for them to lay their eggs. Secondly, we have cage-free hens. In this system, all the birds are free in an aviary.

Reasonably, the majority might deduce that living without a cage (however comfortable and spacious the cage may be) gives hens a better quality of life. On this premise, the British organisation Compassion in Animal Farming [76] launched a campaign to eradicate the use of cages (any type of cage for any animal species) within the European Union. The campaign, called End the Cage Age [77] collected 1.4 million signatures (given the EU has a population of more than 450 million, it doesn't seem to have been very popular). In any case, the EU authorities agreed with the proposal and the use of cages of any kind is to be eliminated by 2027.

What might be more surprising to some readers is that cage-free hens establish strict hierarchies and the most dominant peck and even cannibalise the hens at the bottom. Furthermore, intestinal parasites are more common in cage-free systems and, in free range systems, it's not uncommon for an animal to end up in the jaws of a predator. In short, in cage-free systems more hens are needed to produce the same number of eggs than in an enriched cage system.

The aim of these examples is to show that animal welfare is almost never black and white but a whole range of greys. And that what seems better to us is of little relevance. It's the animals, in this case, hens who have to decide what's better for them.

And how do we know what's important to a hen? Animal welfare experts design studies that allow us to see their preferences. For example: How do we know how important laying eggs in a nest is to hens [78]? In this example, a bird was put in a space with food and water and a very narrow access to a nest. This access was made more difficult over time, and this allowed researchers to measure the effort hens would make to access the nest and thus how important it was to the animal. This study showed that access to the nest was more important than having litter to scratch, as the effort made for the latter was less than for the former. We can compare preferences. This enables us to conclude that one productive system is not always better than another and that assuming that eliminating one of them is a panacea does not match the reality.

Let's take another example: we have two dogs that live in two different houses, and both want to go out. In one case, the owner doesn't let the dog go out and waits to take it out at the usual time – on a lead. After all, there are vehicles on the roads that could injure the animal, there are strangers who could attack the dog, or other uncontrolled dogs could bite it. In the other case, the owner does let it go out. The dog wants to run and the exercise is good for it, meeting other dogs is a good way of socialising and being with its own kind, and digging and sniffing trees where other dogs have urinated is very beneficial for the dog. The two owners love their dogs but which cares more and best for their welfare? There isn't a correct answer and there are a lot of caveats to consider.

Firstly, on some occasions welfare involves finding a balance between different animals that live in the same farm. Consider lactating sows for example. A few days before the birth and until they have finished nursing their piglets (around 30 days in total), in some farms the sows are confined to metal cages that prevent them from walking and turning around. This is not the result of a desire to harm the sow or to fatten it by preventing it from moving or anything like that. The reason is simple: when a loose sow throws itself to the ground, it often squashes a piglet.

The cages allow the sow to lie down but it must do so more slowly. This gives the young piglets, which are still clumsy, time to move to a safe spot and thus prevents numerous deaths by asphyxiation. This example shows that welfare is not an absolute value and can impact different animals on the same farm in different ways. The farmers who prefer to use systems that don't restrict the movement of the sow have a

It must be the science and not the perception of certain organisations that determines what is welfare and what isn't

higher piglet mortality rate [79]. Do the people demanding the elimination of cages for all species know this?

The evolution of the science of animal welfare could help us solve this and other problems but, in my opinion, it must be the sector and experts who determine what is possible and when. Outside pressure from NGOs and political organisations generally far removed from the agricultural sector can have negative consequences for the exact thing it is trying to improve: animal welfare.

Evidently, knowledge of animal welfare continues to progress, and some systems have been shown to be counter-productive to the correct physical and psychological development of the animals. For example, to continue with hens, battery cages, which were banned in the EU in 2012, did not allow the hens to move or extend their wings. But it must be the science and not the perception of certain organisations that determines what is welfare and what isn't.

In 1986, the Department of Veterinary Medicine of the University of Cambridge appointed Professor Donald Broom as the first ever professor of animal welfare [80]. Since then, every veterinary faculty has incorporated this discipline and it should be them, the people who know about the subject, who determine – or at least try to determine – what welfare is for each animal, how it can be realistically optimised in a way that allows the farmer to remain competitive and the public to continue enjoying accessible animal products in their shopping basket.

And here we come to a key point where animals demonstrate a preference for being in a confined system rather than in the wild. The scientist and pioneer of the study of animal welfare William Thorpe explained this in one of his most well-known works [81].

In it, he describes how African buffaloes had to be moved to another region because there were too many animals in their home region. They were stabled for a time during this process. Once freed for reintroduction into the wild, they clearly showed a desire to go back into the stables, particularly at night. The buffaloes had experienced life in the wild and life on a farm and preferred the latter. Ultimately, having food guaranteed and being out of the reach of lions and other predators was worth sacrificing some freedom for. Other authors have described similar experiences [71]. It's very possible that this behaviour was there at the start of the domestication of many species.

Nevertheless, it's vital that farmers understand that this isn't *carte blanche* to remove all freedom from their animals, to pay no consideration to their animals' welfare. This is unfortunately the case in some countries that, for example, still allow laying hens to be farmed in battery cages – where the hens cannot extend their wings or turn around – that are objectively harmful to the welfare of these birds. It is therefore important to insist that European legislation in this area is the strictest in the world and is in constant evolution to adapt to new scientific knowledge, and contains requirements that farmers must meet covering all the aspects that are important for the animals – according to species – and their welfare: the availability of space, drinking troughs, management practices, air quality, type of floor, and many more.

In general, for an animal to be productive, it must be in good health given that disease and stress have a negative effect on

We must remember that the farmers are the people most interested in their animals producing to their maximum capabilities. And, in general, for an animal to be productive, it must be in good health given that disease and stress have a negative effect on productivity. There are cases in which this rule isn't a hundred percent true [82] but farmers know that improvements in welfare will result in healthy animals that produce more.

There are livestock farming practices that, from an urban perspective, are hard to accept without the appropriate context. For example, dehorning calves shortly after birth is necessary to prevent the injuries to people and other animals that would be certain to occur if the animals' horns developed fully.

Another process that can be shocking is cutting the tails (tail docking) of sheep and pigs. There are good (animal welfare) reasons for the practice. Sheep that retain their tails accumulate more dirt in their hindquarters, which can attract flies whose larvae feed on the animals' skin. Piglets, if they keep their tails, have the bad habit of biting one another, causing injury and infection. To round off these examples, we'll mention beak trimming, which is sometimes practised on laying birds at a few days of age to prevent them pecking one another and causing serious injuries and to prevent undesirable behaviour, such as cannibalism [83].

All these practices must be carried out with anaesthesia, and anti-inflammatory medicines that alleviate the pain should be administered. Sometimes these practices may not be performed (e.g. tail docking of piglets) and farmers may try to minimise the negative impact with other techniques, such as reducing stocking densities, changing diets and even adding toys such as balls, to the stalls to keep the animals distracted.

We have to remember that, like all science, animal welfare is also progressing. Until not that long ago, dairy cows' tails were routinely docked on a lot of farms as it was thought that because they were dirty, they made the animals more likely to suffer mastitis (a consequence of a mammary gland infection). However, over time it was demonstrated that this practice had no scientific basis and today it has been eliminated.

It should be pointed out that extensive systems are not necessarily better than intensive systems when it comes to animal welfare. That's because, even though they allow the animals to move more and express other behaviours, it also exposes them to negative factors that could affect their quality of life, such as attacks from predators or inclement weather.

In fact, intensive and industrial systems can offer animals high levels of welfare, as has been demonstrated by numerous studies [84] [85] [86]. Indeed, in the event of epidemics in wild animals, the health of animals on extensive farms with access to the outside world may suffer because they are more likely to come into contact with wild animals [87]. Bird flu, present in wild migratory birds, is a paradigmatic example. When it appears, birds on extensive farms have to stay inside to avoid being infected.

Therefore, we can conclude that living in the wild does not prevent suffering and that, while production systems can cause discomfort and may not offer perfect welfare, they enable the animals to be fed, protected against predators, and sheltered. Furthermore, in Europe and other countries, legislation protects them and guarantees their welfare, and they are given veterinary care which, as we have shown, has enabled us to eradicate or contain major diseases that also affect wild animals.

To illustrate this, let's travel to Ethiopia and the year 1888 [88]. An epidemic has broken out among its cattle. Cattle plague has wiped out, in a few weeks, almost every Ethiopian herd. There are no animals left for food or oxen to work the fields. Without their strength, the earth cannot be ploughed and cereals cannot be harvested.

The eradication of African swine fever from Spain is another example of how protecting domesticated livestock also indirectly protects wildlife: in this case, wild boars

Wild ruminants, such as antelopes, giraffes and buffaloes, are also falling victim to the plague. Famine grips the country. The testimony of a French missionary gives an idea of the scale of the disaster: "Everywhere I go I come across walking skeletons or corpses half-eaten by hyenas, corpses of the starving who have died of exhaustion [89]".

The efforts to prevent cattle plague epidemics, which were common in Europe until the 19th century, present in Asia until the middle of the 20th century and present in Africa until well into the 1980s, meant that various countries found effective prevention. These efforts were rewarded with the elimination, thanks to vaccines, of this disease from the face of the earth in 2011. We can see, therefore, how a global effort to protect livestock also resulted in the protection of wildlife, which clearly, was very susceptible to this virus.

The case of the eradication of African swine fever from Spain is another example of how protecting domesticated livestock also indirectly protects wildlife: in this case, wild boars. And this continues to be relevant today as the virus is once again present in wild pigs in Europe. Vaccines are being developed that will allow us to protect wild boars in order to safeguard the health and welfare of farm animals [90]. We could mention other diseases, such as rabbit haemorrhagic disease, which decimated European and Asian livestock numbers and caused a massive death toll among wild rabbits, which indirectly further endangered the recovery of the lynx by depriving it of its natural prey. The development of vaccines that control the spread of the virus on farms is helping to limit the circulation of the virus in the wild [91] [92].

Another very illustrative example comes from fish farming. In this case, farming activity has saved some wild species. Since the end of the 1980s, the number of wild fish being caught has remained at the same level. Today we eat more fish bred on fish farms than captured by fishing fleets [93]. This is great news for the environment and marine fishing grounds.

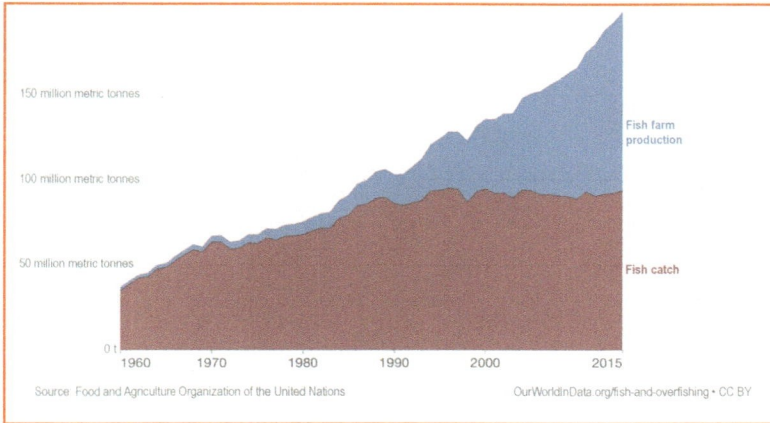

Evolution of wild fish and farmed fish consumption. Today we eat more farmed than wild fish. Acquaculture contributes to the preservation of marine environment

Contrary to what a lot of vegan influencers have published [94], intensive livestock farming is less exposed to infections from wildlife [95], because the isolation and strict controls within the production units to make it much more difficult for pathogens to get in and out.

We can't ignore the fact that the presence of a lot of animals on large farms creates a risk of viruses or bacteria multiplying rapidly. It's easier for a virus to reproduce rapidly in a barn with fifty thousand chickens than in an aviary with five birds. But it's nonetheless true that the majority of farms provide veterinary care and have equipment for detecting and stemming epidemics. Firstly, they are protected from the outside world; it's hard

JUAN PASCUAL

for wild animals to get in. Furthermore, in many intensive systems the farm workers must shower and put on clothes that they only wear on the farm to prevent any external pathogens from getting in or out. If a virus gets in despite the precautions, as has been the case with outbreaks of bird flu [96], the farm is immediately isolated and the animals sacrificed. For some diseases, this is even required by the legislation [97]. In such cases, the on-farm cases act as sentinels to contain the pathogen and prevent spreading. This is of course made possible by the fact that many of today's farms have highly qualified veterinary teams ready to respond to any infectious diseases.

Epidemics since 1900 that caused more than one thousand deaths.

Source: Juan Pascual. Adapted from https://en.wikipedia.org/wiki/List_of_epidemics

The fact is that the vast majority of pandemics involving animals originated either in livestock living with families with the resulting complete lack of sanitary control, or in hunting. In large parts of Asia, Africa and Latin America, it is common for families to keep a few birds at home or in a pen, living with them. This has been a very important focus in several flu epidemics. In contrast, modern farms require few workers, which massively reduces the possiblity of bird-human contact.

Primate hunting was the vector that brought the AIDS virus into contact with humans [98] and Ebola reached our species as a result of hunting apes and bats [99]. This latter species appears to be the cause of the origin of the coronavirus Covid-19 pandemia

The three diseases (AIDS, Ebola, coronavirus) originated in countries with limited resources and complex and very expensive access to meat (China was in the middle of an African swine fever crisis that had forced the country to sacrifice hundreds of millions of pigs at the time of Covid-19). In places where buying meat is easy, as it is in countries with significant livestock herds, there is no need to hunt and to come into contact with species that could be carrying pathogenic viruses. For the reasons mentioned above, we can deduce that livestock protects us from pandemics rather than causing them. A person who can buy a chicken for a decent price doesn't go out hunting monkeys or bats.

Indeed, we shouldn't forget that one of the most devastating infectious diseases in history, smallpox, which was responsible for 300 million deaths in the 20th century alone and has now been eradicated, was first prevented thanks to cows (hence the name vaccine from the Latin word vacca for cow). The virus that affected cows caused a mild disease in humans and made them immune to human smallpox. The frequent contact that shepherds and dairy farmers had with cows gave them protection. The British doctor Edward Jenner observed this phenomenon and used the animal virus to protect humans [100], saving millions of lives. So, to date, rather than being the source of pandemics, livestock farming seems to have prevented them.

Intensive livestock farming is less exposed to infections from wildlife, because the isolation and strict controls in the production units make it much more difficult for pathogens to get in and out

The production of animals for slaughter, especially in the West, acts as a factor in keeping the animal population in rural areas and, as such, helps to protect them from urban rapacity or migration to the cities. Faced with the accusing finger of animal rights activists against livestock farming, which in their view is guilty of being the source of all the planet's ills from climate change to eutrophication in the Gulf of Mexico to deforestation, we can see that not everything is black and white, and that livestock farming not only makes very positive contributions to the environment but also to the food security of billions of people, and to the hundreds of industries that use its products.

We see, therefore, that there are deep links between human societies and the animals that live with them, a link that shapes

71

the former and has led to the evolution of the latter. This link provides significant benefits for both parties, but some people want to break it. We will analyse their reasons and arguments, and the responses we can give to their claims.

.

REASONS
FOR ANIMAL
RIGHTS

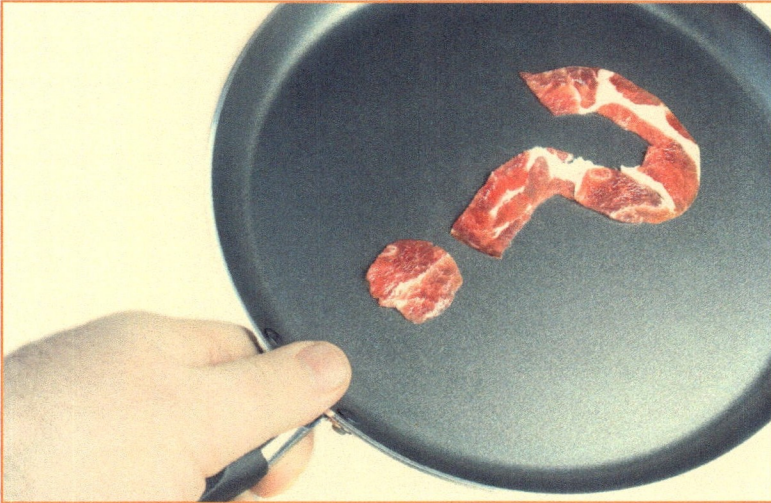

People who embrace animal rights activism or veganism do so for a variety of reasons, the most common of which are:

1   Ethical reasons. With caveats, an animal rights activist's reasoning would be that slaughtering an animal and ending the life of a sentient being is bad. Even if the animal is not slaughtered – as is the case in egg, milk and wool production – its life in a stable is pitiful and, therefore, consuming these products encourages an industry that vegans want no part of.

2   A not insignificant number defend their choice as an act of defence of the environment because, they argue, the production of animal products uses huge amounts of resources and contributes to the deterioration of the environment, which they claim would not happen with plant-based diets.

3   Another reason vegans put forward is health. This is the most common motivation, with 42% of new vegans giving this reason in surveys [101].

4   Lastly, we have those who choose this option simply for religious reasons. This is the case for some Hindu denominations, although in this case they are vegetarians and not strict vegans as they are allowed to consume dairy products.

This means that eating meat is not negative *in itself* for the majority of the vegan community. I'll explain. Some of the companies researching how to produce lab-grown meat or other alternatives to animal products are funded or run by vegan patrons [102]. This is also the case with companies aiming to produce milk from genetically modified yeast. So, if artificial meat doesn't have the aforementioned problems (clearly 1 would be solved, it's not so clear that 2 would be), eating this type of meat would be perfectly acceptable from a vegetarian perspective.

Let's take another example to illustrate this point:

if a cow is struck by lightning, its death would be completely accidental and would have nothing to do with its owners. Therefore, from an animal rights perspective there would be no reason not to eat it. This would also be the case for meat produced in a laboratory (if it ever becomes a reality, which is highly doubtful).

Roadkill may seem a somewhat far-fetched example, but less so when we see that, in fact, there are vegan groups that allow the eating of roadkill. In other words, the eating of animals that have been run over on the road [103]. Some consider this meat to be the most ethical meat (even as the only ethical way of eating meat and see doing so a moral duty [104]) and there is a growing movement encouraging its consumption, as proven by the numerous websites dedicated to recipes for roadkill on the internet.

Even more far-fetched, but no less true, is the consumption of human placenta recommended by some vegans [105]. The placenta is the organ that provides nutrients to the foetus in the womb. After the birth, it is eliminated naturally. A lot of animals, including herbivores, eat the placenta after the birth, possibly to prevent the organic waste attracting predators. The US actress Mayim Bialik, who played Sheldon Cooper's frustrated girlfriend in the series *The Big Bang Theory*, claims to have eaten her own placenta. The actress is a known animal rights activist [106], and claims that if animals eat their own placenta it's because we have evolved to do so. Clearly the fact that our teeth and digestive system have evolved for a diet that includes meat doesn't seem to have had any effect on her militancy.

In principle, there shouldn't be any problem eating the eggs, drinking the milk or wearing the wool of an animal whose welfare has not been negatively affected. Even Peter Singer, the guru of the vegan movement and author of the best-seller *Animal Liberation* accepts this possibility [107]. However, the majority of animal rights activists do not consider the use of any animal product to be compatible with the animal's welfare, so they renounce their consumption.

Let's take a look at each of these four aspects in more detail.

I

ETHICAL REASONS.
IS SLAUGHTERING ANIMALS MORAL?

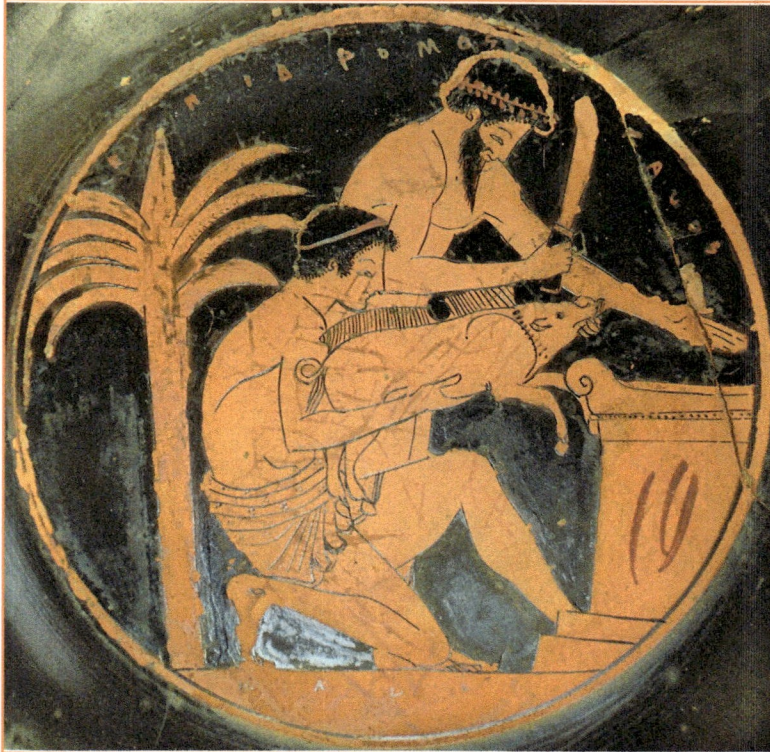

Is taking the life of an animal to eat it or to use it for biomedical research morally justifiable? This is perhaps the most subjective of all the aspects we're going to look at, as there are a wide range of opinions that are all based on debatable criteria and, therefore, far from objective. Nevertheless, we will try to approach the issue from three perspectives:

1   The first will look at the inevitability of some deaths, regardless of the diet we choose.

2 The second will consider the criteria most frequently used by the vegan community to give animals the same moral standing as humans and why, in my opinion, it is wrong to place animals on the same moral plane as us.

3 Finally, the third, eminently practical, will describe what the consequences would be if the world opted, *en masse*, for a vegan diet.

1 IT'S INEVITABLE THAT SOME ANIMALS WILL DIE AS A RESULT OF FOOD PRODUCTION

Let's start with an objective fact: it's inevitable that some animals will die irrespective of the diet we choose. Even following a strict vegan diet does not prevent some animals dying so that we can feed ourselves. The production of vegetables requires the use of pesticides to prevent the harvests being destroyed by insects, snails and rodents. Agricultural machinery destroys bird nests and the dens of small mammals and reptiles that have bred amongst the harvest. So, the first calculation could be a quantitative one: which diet generates fewest deaths? As we will see, there are carnivorous diets that clearly have a smaller impact in terms of the number of deaths than vegan diets.

According to Michael Archer [108], a professor at the University of New South Wales and an expert in biology and environmental sciences, a pasture-raised calf in Australia produces 45 kg of protein (from an original weight of 288 kg, removing the weight of the bones and entrails and considering beef to be approximately 23% protein). In other words, two calves would give us almost 100 kg of high-quality protein to use to feed ourselves. In contrast, in the same country, 100 mice die per hectare as a consequence of the rat poison used so grain can be grown. To obtain 100 kg of wheat protein (wheat is 13% protein), we would need the amount of grain produced on half a hectare (based on production in Australia). In other words, to obtain the same quantity of protein from wheat, 55 mammals, in this case mice, die compared to two calves (if these cows have been pasture-raised). And that's without going into detail about the quality of the protein that beef provides: not only is beef protein much richer in amino acids, it also provides vitamins and minerals that wheat lacks.

This calculation confirms previous studies that reported an 80% decrease in the mice population [109] immediately after the harvesting of a cropped area.

An equivalent approximation, this time with data from the USA, suggests that, if all of the US adopted a vegan diet, 1.8 billion animals would be killed every year by harvesters and other agricultural machinery given that a greater area of land would have to be cultivated to replace products of animal origin [110].

Some authors have questioned the figures these studies have provided [111], but however wrong they are there's no doubt that many more rodents, reptiles and birds (not counting insects, snails and other invertebrates) die when half a hectare of wheat is harvested than if we consume the meat or milk of a pasture-raised cow [112].

This example demonstrates that consuming plants does not preclude animal suffering [113] and that some carnivorous diets involve a lower number of animal deaths than a strict vegetarian diet.

A lot of animals are attracted by plant crops. The Bugs Bunny cartoons show the eternal dispute between the farmer producing the carrots and the animated rabbit's appetite, which is never fully satiated.

But it is not just a funny story, but a totally realistic one that explains why, in a period of five years, 200,000 ducks were shot to protect rice fields in Australia or why, in order to protect pea crops, it is necessary to kill hundreds of deer, possums and kangaroos [114] [115]. Not even fencing off these fields would be enough to avoid a lot of the deaths because it would cut off a lot of routes the animals follow to escape predators, reproduce, and find food.

A closer example would be the deaths of birds as a result of the olive harvest. Once again, it is the machinery that is responsible for the destruction of nests and sucking in thousands of birds [116].

On the other hand, many insects die in the processing of food and cannot be separated. Their presence is so inevitable that

79

US legislation [117] allows a certain amount of insect remains in many foods. So, pasta may contain 225 insect fragments per 225 g of product or a cup of raisins may contain up to 33 fruit fly eggs.

We could add to this list the fact that practically all crops use animal manure as fertiliser. Manure accounts for 50% of all fertilizer used globally – so the "suffering" that livestock farming afflicts on animals is also exploited in this way – and a large part of the fruit we consume is the result of bee pollination. According to some animal rights activists, this is another way in which agriculture is complicit in animal cruelty because the bees are "enslaved" for honey production [118].

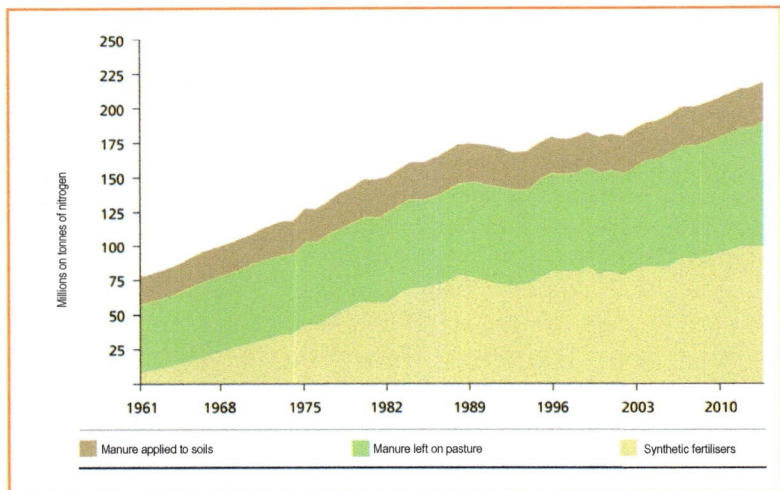

Cumulative global use of nitrogen fertilisers of animal and synthetic origin.
Source: © FAO 2018 Nitrogen inputs to agricultural soils from livestock manure. Page 18 https://www.fao.org/documents/card/en/c/I8153EN.

It is, therefore, clear that eating only a plant-based diet doesn't rule out the need for animals or the possibility that a large number of animals have been harmed to produce the food. As a result, we can conclude that consuming some products from animals bred in a certain way (for example pasture-raised calves) or consuming milk or using wool from animals raised on extensive farms leads to a lower death toll than following a vegan diet.

Other reasons for animal slaughter

We keep on mentioning cases in which it is clear that, for the majority of people, slaughtering an animal is justified and, in fact practically all legal codes recognise that such cases exist. In fact, in many countries there are situations where the slaughtering of animals is not just an option, it is an obligation: animals with certain transmissible infections, such as rabies, must be put down as soon as there is a positive diagnosis [119]. Other diseases result in the immediate slaughter of the animals affected and, in some cases, of the entire farm and even animals on farms within a certain distance.

Recently, we have seen several mink slaughtered due to their susceptibility to COVID-19 in order to protect farmworkers and stop the virus at source.

Evidently, these strict measures aim to protect human health and the health of other animals. In other words, they aim to save both animal and human lives. Recently, we have seen several mink slaughtered due to their susceptibility to COVID-19 in order to protect farmworkers and stop the virus at source [120].

Furthermore, it has also been mandatory on a lot of occasions to slaughter certain animals that represent a risk to public health, for example urban rodents that can transmit severe diseases if their if their population growth is uncontrolled. Such rodents are generally given little attention by animal rights associations (although we should recognise PETA's coherence in mentioning them on its website [121]).

Another example is the importance, in some contexts, of getting rid of invasive species so that native species do not disappear, as we will see in detail below.

However, in most circumstances the decision to kill an animal is based on the capacity we have to take this decision and on placing human life above animal life.

If, as eminent animal rights' theorists and the movements that give them a voice defend, we should respect all sentient creatures, we should abandon practices such as rat extermination and pest control, we should protect invasive species at the cost of local wildlife, we should not kill rabid dogs nor remove parasites from our cats and dogs, not even removing lice or ticks that we may find attached to our skin, since they too are sentient beings.

2. THE PHILOSOPHY BEHIND ANIMAL RIGHTS ACTIVISM. THE MORAL CONSIDERATION OF ANIMALS

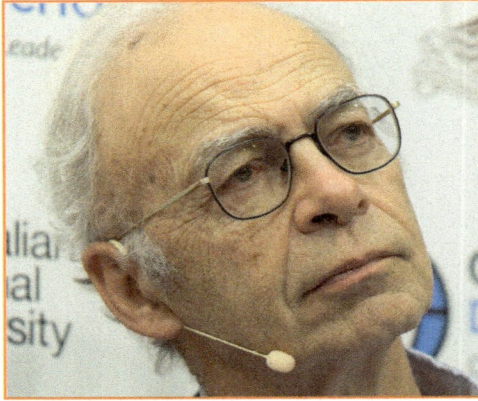

Peter Singer.

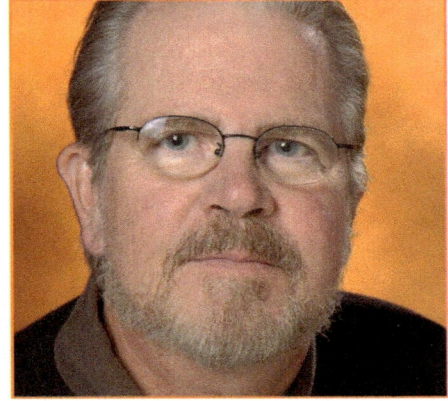

Tom Regan.

However, let's go beyond quantitative reasons and take a look at the qualitative perspective of the arguments put forward against the consumption of meat, eggs, honey, milk and wool, and how we can respond to them. We are entering subjective territory here because the philosophical arguments, although strong, are defenceless against convictions, prejudices and emotions. And, as we have seen, veganism is not particularly sensitive to reasoning, hence it is legally recognised as similar to a religion.

So that we can better understand the scope of an act and determine if it is moral or not, we need to understand that, for the vast majority of philosophers who have studied this question, moral acts are only moral if they are universal [122]. We cannot qualify as moral an action that only benefits the person who performs it; it must be positive for the community as a whole. To illustrate this, let's imagine that tomorrow all the inhabitants of the planet decided unanimously to stop disposing of rubbish, paper or any other waste anywhere other than the designated places. At a stroke we would stop throwing plastics into the sea and paper onto the floor, cigarette butts would disappear from beaches, and we would stop seeing pet faeces on the streets. I think we can agree that this initiative would make the world a better place – cleaner without a doubt – and we would all benefit. This moral act benefits everyone and there are no negative secondary effects.

Let's look, then, at the arguments put forward by the thinkers who have had the greatest influence on animal rights, and therefore vegan, ideology, and let's assess the moral dimension of their proposals.

We'll focus our attention on two philosophers. They're certainly not the only two, and we will mention some others, but they are the thinkers that, without a doubt, laid the foundations of the ideology. The first is Tom Regan and the second, who is even more significant given the media success of his hypotheses, Peter Singer, who we will analyse in greater depth.

The aim here is not to summarise their reasoning – their books and articles are out there – but to get to their root, to explain them, and then respond to them. Both philosophers propose a common element, namely that the capacities for reasoning and self-awareness, which distinguish humans from all other species, should not be considered as a sufficient differentiating element to allow us to use animals for our own benefit.

In other words, the moral community created by and for humans should, according to these authors, also include if not all animals then a significant proportion of them, and that animals should be situated at the same moral level as people, as if they also possessed the capacities that distinguish us as humans.

Based on this common element, Singer and Regan present different arguments. Regan, who was a professor at the University of North Carolina, puts forward a Kantian argument. Kant's categorical imperative claims that humans have an intrinsic value and must not be used as a means to satisfy the aims of others. This principle applies to all humans simply because they are human, even if they lack the capacity to reason, for example people in a vegetative state or very young children. In his own words, we can summarise Kantian thought with regard to animals with this quote: "So far as animals are concerned, we have no direct duties. Animals are not self-conscious and are there merely as the means to an end. That end is man" [123].

Regan disagrees with the Kant because he believes that animals also have intrinsic value (even though, like some disabled humans, they lack the ability to reason) and that animals deserve respect *per se* because, like humans, they are "subjects-of-a-life" and therefore deserve not to be used as a means to our ends. This implies that the same principle that Kant applied to all humans should also apply to animals and, thus, animals should be treated with respect and not be harmed except for cases of *force majeure*.

Regan accepts that the life of a healthy human has more value than the life of an animal because they have an intellectual richness, plans for the future and consciousness that far exceed those of an animal. However, for the same reason, he also considers the life of a healthy dog to be more valuable than that of a severely mentally disabled human or a human in a coma [124]. The same yardstick we apply to people must therefore be applied to animals, at least to those animals which, like birds and mammals, Regan considers "like us to possess a variety of sensory, cognitive and volitional capacities. They see and hear, believe and desire, remember and anticipate, plan and intend. Moreover, what happens to them matters to them. Physical pleasure and pain – these they share with us. But also fear and contentment, anger and loneliness, frustration and satisfaction..." [125].

"It seems the whole world has licence to attribute emotion, empathy, reflection and other human attributes to non-human species, as if there were no limits, as if there were no rules". Marian Dawkins

It's striking how Regan, in addition to his prudent analysis of the rights of animals, describes and attributes sentiments and psychological characteristics to animals although it is far from proven that they possess them. As Marian Dawkins, professor of ethology and animal welfare at the University of Oxford, says "it seems the whole world has licence to attribute emotion, empathy, reflection and other human attributes to non-human species, as if there were no limits, as if there were no rules. As if these were the same attributions in them or in us" [126].

Regan considers the richness of life experience to be of higher quality in healthy people, since they can define their future, remember their past, think abstractly, etc. but he does not think this way in the case of severely mentally handicapped people or sick babies.

To illustrate Regan's position in practice, let's travel back to 1984 for a moment.

That year, a girl was born in the USA with a severe heart problem. The only solution doctors could find to try to save her life was to implant an ape's, specifically a baboon's, heart. It was the first inter-species transplant in history. Sadly, the procedure was not successful and the baby girl, known as Baby Fae, died three weeks after the operation.

Tom Regan published an article [127] in which he claimed that this transplant was an ethical error and that they had not respected the rights of the baboon because he too had a right to life and to not be harmed.

The reader can draw their own conclusions. Personally, I doubt whether the author would have written the article (published a year after Baby Fae's death) if the child had survived or if she had been close to the author.

What the American philosopher wanted to do was to present to us a contradiction, namely: if we use animals for experiments based on their lack of reasoning, we should be ready to use comatose people for this purpose too because their rationality is much lower than that of a healthy animal.

Let's leave Tom Regan for now and analyse in detail the position of the other big animal rights guru, the Australian philosopher Peter Singer, who is without doubt the movement's most influential thinker. He is the philosopher we will mention the most and whose theories we will question the most. In his magnum opus *Animal Liberation* [128], Singer argues that it is not human intellectual capacity that should guide moral consideration to others but their capacity to suffer. Thus, he added to and developed the thesis of the English philosopher Jeremy Bentham, considered the father of utilitarianism, whose objective was to achieve the "greatest happiness for the greatest number". The word number includes any sentient being. In fact, for Bentham, the question that determines whether individuals are moral is not 'can they reason?', nor 'can they talk?' but 'can they suffer?'. This belief, nevertheless, didn't stop Bentham from eating meat whenever he wanted to [129].

Let's pause for a moment and review Singer's utilitarian philosophical vision (also known as consequentialism) [130]. Utilitarianism considers actions to be moral or immoral based on their consequences. So, we must choose the action that gives the greatest satisfaction or results in the least harm. We will give two examples that illustrate this school of thought's thesis: imagine we're in a railway signalling box. A convoy is out of control and approaching a set of points. There are five workers on the track that it is currently heading towards. On the other track, there is only one. If we follow this philosophical doctrine, we should change the points so that the train does the least possible amount of damage and runs over one worker not five.

This example clearly shows the good intentions of this doctrine but appearances can be deceiving. Applying "mathematics" to morality can lead us to perverse conclusions: let's suppose five people need an organ transplant to survive: two need a kidney transplant, one a heart transplant, one a liver transplant, and one a lung transplant. We might think that it's worth sacrificing one healthy young person to get these organs. After all, we'll cut short one life, but we'll save the lives of five people. I don't think it's necessary to explain how repugnant this action would be from an ethical perspective. This is why utilitarianism is questioned by numerous philosophers [131].

Even Regan himself rejects this philosophy. Here, the two thinkers disagree, I would say clash, because, as Regan explains, if a gang rapes a person, the potential satisfaction of the rapists may be greater, quantitatively, than the humiliation, pain and anger of the victim. Therefore, according to utilitarians, this action could be positive if we weigh up the pleasure and suffering [132].

Therefore, for Singer's philosophy what confers moral status to an individual is not their capacity to reason but rather their capacity to experience pleasure or pain. That's because, according to Singer, the capacity to suffer is the indispensable prerequisite for having interests and, in his view, the same interests deserve the same consideration. If a being suffers, no matter their intellectual level, there's no reason not to take this suffering into consideration.

In his own words: "To have interests, in a strict, nonmetaphorical sense, a being must be capable of suffering or experiencing pleasure. If a being suffers, there can be no moral justification for disregarding that suffering, or for refusing to count it equally with the like suffering of any other being." Another quote: "The capacity for suffering and enjoyment is a prerequisite for having interests at all, a condition that must be satisfied before we can speak of interests in a meaningful way." We will see later how plants also have interests even though, as far as we know, they do not have the capacity to suffer or feel pleasure.

It's about finding an appropriate balance so that we can benefit from animal products and that they also benefit by having a life in which they can behave naturally without the scarcity and stress that are an inevitably part of life in the wild.

Furthermore, we could argue that, according to Singer's thesis, if genetic engineering enabled us to create cows and pigs that don't feel pain, we would then be permitted to eat them [133]. Would that be an ethical development? Would it be OK to create animals without a brain and without a personality in order to produce animal products? In my opinion, the respect that animals deserve should push us towards adapting farming systems to their natural behaviour. It's not a question of simply farming without any consideration for the animals or of abolishing animal production. It's about finding an appropriate balance so that we can benefit from animal products and that they also benefit by having a life in which they can behave naturally without the scarcity and stress that are an inevitable part of life in the wild. There is no doubt that an animal that is unable to behave as its species does naturally would be saved from suffering but it would also lose pleasures and positive sensations that, certainly, it still experiences on a farm.

Singer claims that, just as we shouldn't discriminate against a woman for her sex, and that doing so would be a form of discrimination called sexism, nor against a person of a different ethnicity because that would be a form of exclusion we call racism, we should also not discriminate against an animal because it has less cognitive capacity or a lower intellectual level, because that would be a form of exclusion known as speciesism (a term widely used in animal rights jargon and coined by the psychologist Richard D. Ryder in 1970 [134], although it was Singer who popularised it in his book *Animal Liberation*).

Given that what should guide our moral behaviour towards someone is not their cognitive capacities but their capacity to suffer and, since animals can suffer, it would therefore follow that they deserve the same moral consideration as people. Therefore, if we use an irrational animal for experiments based on the argument that their consciousness is less developed than ours, as a logical consequence we should accept experimenting on humans in a vegetative state. As this would repulse the majority of us, Singer concludes that subjecting animals to our productive or experimental processes should also repulse us and that, if this is not the case, we are committing an act of subjective discrimination that the animal rights movement, as we have seen, calls speciesism.

Using animals as food or in experiments with the aim of improving the lives of humans should not be morally questionable, especially if their life has been lived in a state of good welfare and they have also been able to have positive experiences.

Now that we have explained the nucleus of these two authors' ideas, we can respond to them and highlight aspects of their arguments that contain errors, contradictions and significant omissions.

The first contradiction is that both authors claim that the moral consideration does not depend on reasoning but on the intrinsic value of the animal's life (Regan) or their capacity to suffer (Singer). However, unintentionally both thinkers open the door to the following interpretation: moral consideration *does* depend on rationality and the less rational the animal is, the less consideration the animal deserves, regardless of its species. After all, it is intelligence that determines the extent of the capacity to suffer or feel pleasure (all the information we have suggests that a beached whale suffers more than a clam dug up from the sand).

It seems nonsensical to state one thing (moral consideration should be independent of intelligence) and the opposite (a person in vegetative state does not deserve the same moral consideration as a healthy animal) and claim to be right on both occasions.

Singer also falls into other contradictions, If he wants to end livestock farming because, according to him, it causes pain and discomfort for the animals, he should also consider that the animals also experience well-being and pleasure since they are given food, don't have any predators, can play with animals of their species (in some farms), etc. Furthermore, we should also consider the benefit of those who consume their products, many of whom don't have alternative sources of proteins, and of those who benefit from animal testing conducted to develop medicines. Why does he not centre his discourse on optimising welfare rather than centring it exclusively on eliminating pain? [135]. The first approach would lead us to improving farms and experiments; the second, which Singer has opted for, to eliminating them.

But let's look at a profound philosophical aspect that's not necessarily easy to objectify. Is taking the life of an animal to eat it or to use it for scientific experiments morally justifiable? With regard to this point, I want to start by pointing out that every legal system in the world and all past and present societies have valued human life over animal life.

Why is a human worthy of greater moral consideration than a living being that, although lacking rationality or at least lacking rationality compared to humans, still feels and can suffer? What are legislators' reasons for giving human life this pre-eminence? Why, in my opinion, are Singer's and Regan's arguments erroneous?

Firstly, because the life of a healthy human (and both philosophers agree on this point) is of more value than, let's say, that of a mouse. Unlike animals – at least, according to our current knowledge of them – human beings plan their future, have self-awareness, are capable of overcoming their instincts, possess a rich language, develop institutions, question their position in the universe, the transcendence of their lives and, above all, collaborate with and anticipate the reactions of fellow members of their species. They also transmit a culture to future generations. That's why a human life is more valuable than the life of an animal. And to reiterate, both authors agree with this point [128].

So, if all animals and all humans exhibit the differences listed above, and provided that animals have been raised with adequate welfare conditions and are slaughtered painlessly, there is no reason to object to their use as food. It is true that when we slaughter them we cut short their life. However, as we have seen, their existence is of less value and, therefore, using them as food or in experiments with the aim of improving the lives of humans should not be morally questionable, especially if their life has been lived in a state of good welfare and they have also been able to have positive experiences.

Note that both Regan and Singer would agree with me if I agreed that I would be willing to give the same treatment to a mentally disabled human with equivalent (or less) sensitivity to an animal.

In other words, the reason they are against the way society uses animals is not that they cannot be the object of experiments, but that society is not willing to conduct these same experiments on humans. They call this position speciesist. In reality, it's not. If, for example, there were an alien civilisation we could communicate with and the members of this civilisation had brain activity similar to ours – they planned their future, they passed on a culture and were fully aware of their surroundings – this civilisation and its members would deserve the same consideration as humans even though they were from a species genetically far removed from ours. The same would be true if we found some lost Neanderthals on a remote island. They would be genetically different but, as far as we know, their intellectual activity would be similar to ours.

> Singer claims that "killing a snail or a day-old infant does not thwart any desires of this kind (i.e., desires for the future), because snails and newborn infants are incapable of having such desires".

The problem Singer presents us with, is that of interests. In other words, it's not the animal's level of consciousness that's important but rather their capacity to suffer. Hence, he explains that the capacity to suffer or feel pleasure is a prerequisite for having interests. A stone cannot have interests because it doesn't suffer or feel pleasure. Therefore, these capacities are not only necessary, they are sufficient to say that an animal has an interest in avoiding suffering. And it's that capacity to suffer (and therefore the obligation to avoid it) that makes a living being a moral entity and grants it a moral status.

We can offer counterarguments to Singer and Regan with similar reasoning for both philosophers since, even though their philosophies differ (capacity to suffer and intrinsic value, respectively), the following arguments provide a response to both:

Singer claims that "killing a snail or a day-old infant does not thwart any desires of this kind (i.e., desires for the future), because snails and newborn infants are incapable of having such desires" [136].

When giving the life of a newborn baby the same status as that of a snail, Singer seems to ignore the fact that a baby has potential that an animal does not, as a baby will become an adult whose life will be much richer than that of any other animal. The interests of the people who love the baby and whose feelings, relationships and empathy, which do not have a parallel in the relationships that the snails may have with each other or the social life the snails may develop, should also be taken into account. The baby lives in a society that considers it a member of that society and, for that very reason, it is not indifferent to what is happening. This aspect marks a decisive qualitative difference *in nature and not only in degree* compared to the animal world.

Both philosophers insist on the possibility of experimenting on people in a vegetative state. After all, their life is much less rich than that of a healthy adult, and even that of a healthy mouse. Furthermore, as they are human, the results of the experiments would be almost immediately applicable to the population as a whole. So if we accept medical testing on a mouse, why shouldn't we conduct testing on someone in a persistent vegetative state.

We can answer this by stating that there are cases of people in a vegetative state who have recovered. Of course, it's not common but we have all read news articles about people who have recovered their former level of consciousness after spending years in a coma. Therefore, given the possibility of a potential recovery, it would be morally reprehensible to experiment on such a subject [137].

On the other hand, the fact that a person's mental faculties are irreversibly impaired does not make them less valuable to their family or to society as a whole. A person who suffers an accident that leaves them disabled is not loved any less by their family as a result and, in the vast majority of cases, the family would refuse to allow their loved one's body to be used for experiments. This is because the feelings the person's fellow human beings have for them are based on what they are – a human being – and not on the level of their mental capabilities [138]. As animals lack these sentiments for members of their species in such circumstances, we can state that human beings,

91

however disabled they are, have value for others and, therefore, deserve respect for who they are.

Furthermore, thanks to social networks – we could even say from the moment we invented writing – humans are sharing information with the whole world. Certainly if a human being in a vegetative state were used for experiments, the experiment would be widely criticised and many people would be indignant, which would not happen with animals, oblivious as they are to the fate of the fellow members of their species. Is this yet more proof of speciesism? Not necessarily; a lot of people also protest against animal cruelty. What we still haven't seen is animals protesting against cruelty to fellow members of their species or defending their rights.

The fact that a person's mental faculties are irreversibly impaired does not make them less valuable to their family or to society as a whole.

Lastly, we could all suffer an accident or severe disease that leaves us disabled but the vast majority of us, in full use of our faculties, would be opposed to being used for experiments because our rights as a citizen should not be diminished as a consequence of our diminished capacities [139].

Both philosophers skirt around the issue of religious sentiment. I agree with them that the morality of acts should be argued in a human context – we need to remember the universality of moral acts and that they should be moral for believers and non-believers. However, this doesn't allow us to ignore the fact that billions of people do have faith and that for the majority of them human life is more valuable. Therefore, they would view experiments on humans in a persistent vegetative state with genuine horror.

There is another argument that tears down Singer's assertion. If, as he claims, the life of a person with all their faculties is richer and, therefore, more valuable than that of other animals and deserves greater moral consideration, we should also establish this scale among species. In other words, a mouse would have greater moral consideration than an intestinal worm, seeing how everything suggests that the life of the former is more active, and contains more stimuli and richness than that of the latter.

In fact, Singer himself establishes this difference because he claims that the loss of the ability to feel and, therefore, the moral consideration linked to this feeling occurs somewhere between crustaceans and molluscs [140]. Now, as we have shown, nothing indicates that molluscs, worms and even some unicellular organisms lack the capacity to feel pain.

But there's a more dangerous drift. If the capacity to have a richer, and therefore more valuable life, is linked to the capacity to suffer, in turn linked to intellectual capacity, we can conclude that this latter influences, perhaps even determines, moral consideration. We, therefore, could find human beings who, because they have different mental capabilities, deserve to belong to different moral levels. Thus, people with a higher IQ would have greater moral consideration than, let's say, someone of low intelligence, which would lead us to unjust, undesirable and immoral discrimination.

Furthermore, if the capacity to feel pain is what defines moral consideration, would an anaesthetised animal or person or someone with congenital analgesia (inability to feel pain) not have moral consideration? [141]. And why should it be pain that determines whether or not a being belongs to the moral community? We will delve deeper into this point later.

Morality is the fruit of humans for the sake of humanity [142]. Only humans can have the ability to attribute to themselves this concept which allows us to behave in a way other than that dictated by our instincts, because it is only humans that have, understand and develop the concepts of good and evil. Therefore, we have the capacity to control our instincts and effectively have freedom of choice, which is a virtue missing from the animal world.

If the capacity to feel pain is what defines moral consideration, would an anaesthetised animal or person or someone with congenital analgesia (inability to feel pain) not have moral consideration?

People have intellectual qualities and the ability to collaborate with others that separate us from other species. It's striking to see how animal rights activists disdain human intellectual supremacy as a moral reference but, on the other hand, they try to find references from sciences such as ethology and psychology that would enable them to find these same intellectual qualities (even very rudimentary versions) in other species to thus justify their inclusion in the moral community.

A key difference – we will have opportunity to discuss it in much more detail later – can be found in the fact that belonging to the human species is not limited to having a set of unique mental skills but also manifests in the way we interact as a community. So, for example, people react to murder with laws that punish the killer, not only for taking the life of the victim but also because of how this act affects all of us. In other words, other human beings expect particular behaviour from me – for example that I do not kill my fellow humans – and what humans expect from me, walruses do not expect from their peers.

Therefore, the expectations of our fellow citizens are, in addition to our capacities, also what make us human.

We could even go further. As we have seen, there is a growing interest among certain vegan communities in consuming roadkill – some consider it an obligation. But no one would even consider eating the meat of a person who was the victim of a traffic accident. Why? Because the moral consideration a human cadaver deserves from us is different to that which an animal cadaver deserves. Because with a person – even if we don't know them – we could have shared an ideology, shared secrets, fallen in love, talked, studied, cried, argued or gone to court with them.

Belonging to the human species is not limited to having a set of unique mental skills but also manifests in the way we interact as a community.

Activities, experiences that we can only share with our equals, and which mean that we form a moral community that makes us different to the rest of the animal kingdom. Could we have this type of interaction with other species? It's very possible that we have had, since we all have genetic markers from Neanderthals, which proves that our ancestors reproduced with them [143]. However, they were a species with similar intellectual capacity, with self-awareness, whose life had content and was, therefore, similar value to ours.

Let's look a little more deeply at attitudes of respect towards the cadavers of our fellow humans. It's a behaviour that we find in all cultures and that is supported by legislation all over the world [144] [145]. Even the Geneva Convention requires that cadavers of enemy combatants are buried according to the religion they belonged to [146].

To illustrate this, we can use the example of the "Human Bodies" travelling exhibition, which exhibits plastinated – an anatomical preservation technique that substitutes natural fluids with other fluids to prevent tissue from decaying – cadavers and that has received a lot of criticism following its latest stop in Barcelona [147]. A lot of people are repulsed by the public exhibition of cadavers, some of them in acrobatic postures, for example one of the bodies is shown ready to kick a football.

Recently the rector of a Paris university had to respond to accusations of negligence and a lack of care with regard to the cadavers kept at his institution for classes. Some of them were found in a state of putrefaction and with rodent bites, and there was also a suspicion that body parts were being traded, etc. [148]

But these cases pale in comparison to the social impact and revulsion generated by the case of David Fuller, an electrician who worked in a British hospital morgue who, over the course of more than a decade, used the corpses of at least a hundred women to satisfy his sexual perversions. And if that wasn't enough, he recorded his acts on video [149].

Animals themselves do not have respect for cadavers, nor do we feel the need to treat their cadavers in the same way.

That's because it's not just our intellectual capacities that make us human, it's also our relationships with other people, with our fellow humans. Thus, a person in a persistent vegetative state or a handicapped baby is also the fruit of human love; they have been in their mother's womb for nine months, and they have been raised by and belong to a family. This latter creates a level of intimacy and dependency – and therefore moral meaning – that does not have a parallel in any other species. These relationships that we establish and that we can only establish with our equals dictate that we do not eat our dead or the amputated limbs of our peers, and that we respect their bodies after they have died [150] [151].

We could always argue that, even if a human being has diminished mental capacities, this does not mean that they don't exist, rather it means that they are not being manifest [152]. Therefore, it's easy to understand that if, as a consequence of suffering advanced Alzheimer's disease, a human loses their most basic mental capacities, they will continue to be a father, mother, brother and friend who should be respected, held close and talked to, even if they don't understand us. It will be their hand that we will hold onto to transmit our feelings, it will be, in short, a being with whom we have shared – and can continue to share – human experiences that cannot be transferred outside the community that we humans form.

A person doesn't lose their human condition because they lose their capacities or because they stop feeling pleasure or pain. In his most famous book Singer claims, as we mentioned earlier, that there is an imaginary line somewhere between a shrimp and an oyster [128] at which the capacity to feel stops being present. This line is, of course, totally arbitrary but if it wasn't the Australian philosopher's reasoning would be: a person with Alzheimer's does not suffer and does not feel pleasure, so therefore they are outside all moral consideration (given that moral consideration comes from the ability to feel pleasure or suffer). Therefore, following this reasoning, we could therefore conclude that a person suffering a disease of this type becomes, from a moral perspective, a mollusc. They would belong to the moral catalogue of molluscs – if such a thing existed. Clearly, this conclusion is not only absurd, it is also an ignominy for the people who suffer these diseases and for their families.

> A person in a vegetative state or a handicapped baby is also the fruit of human love; they have been in their mother's womb for nine months and belong to a family. This creates a level of intimacy and dependency – and moral meaning – that does not have a parallel in any other species.

However, there's more. Singer is an open defender of infanticide in cases in which a newborn baby suffers serious diseases such as haemophilia or Down's syndrome. In his own words:

"When the death of a disabled infant will lead to the birth of another infant with better prospects of a happy life, the total amount of happiness will be greater if the disabled infant is killed. The loss of the happy life for the first infant is outweighed by the gain of a happier life for the second. Therefore, if killing the haemophiliac infant has no adverse effect on others, it would, according to the total view, be right to kill him" [122].

Or in other words, the life a haemophiliac baby (who, as an adult, will have the same intellectual level as any other baby) is worth less than the life of a healthy hamster.

Evidently, a priori, nothing indicates that a haemophiliac baby or a baby with Down's syndrome cannot have a happy life and make the people around them happy. Nor can anyone guarantee that

96

killing a child will lead to the birth of another or that this new baby will be perfectly healthy. Furthermore, where do we draw the line between those who should live and those who should die? After all, there are significant variations between different people with Down's syndrome.

Pronouncing so flippantly on the life and death of children with serious illnesses has meant that Singer is not very welcome in Germany, a country with a tragic history of applying eugenics [153] [154].

In this regard, the letter that a lawyer and disability rights activist, who herself had been severely disabled since birth, wrote to Singer is very moving. I will quote some lines from the first paragraph that explain, in all its crudeness, the true face of the Australian philosopher's ideology [155]:

"He insists he doesn't want to kill me. He simply thinks it would have been better, all things considered, to have given my parents the option of killing the baby I once was, and to let other parents kill similar babies as they come along and thereby avoid the suffering that comes with lives like mine and satisfy the reasonable preferences of parents for a different kind of child…".

It should be added that Singer is against the use of taxes to care for disabled babies [156]. You can't deny that he is coherent in his thinking.

His comparisons between newborn babies and snails, who as we have seen he grants similar moral consideration, don't leave anybody indifferent [157] [158].

The aim here is not to create a corollary of animal rights philosophy but to show that this way of thinking, rather than humanising animals, bestialises people.

In addition to his position on animals and people with disabilities, for whom as we have already seen he defends infanticide, the Australian philosopher, the undisputed figurehead of the anti-speciesist movement who presents himself on his website as the "world's most influential living philosopher" [159], is also permissive of sexual relations with animals [160] and with cadavers [161]. In fact, he does not reject any practice at all – there are no limits – if the consequences are not negative [162]. He has also defended the possibility of raping people with certain mental disabilities [163]. This means he elicits a reaction but having this academic as your standard bearer is more than a little questionable; it doesn't exactly reinforce the animal rights movement's empathic aspect.

If, according to anti-speciesists, excluding animals from all moral consideration due to their lower cognitive abilities is arbitrary, I don't see how claiming that moral consideration should be based on the capacity to suffer or feel pleasure is any less arbitrary. We could make an absurd argument but nonetheless a valid – and arbitrary – one that only living beings capable of understanding the beauty of works of art [164] or the offside rule in football should be granted moral consideration.

If the capacity to feel pain is the north star that defines membership or not of the moral community, we could argue that worms are part of it since they are able to learn how to avoid unpleasant sensations.

Nevertheless, Singer claims that the capacity to feel pain is the factor that determines interests (interest in not suffering or in feeling pleasure) but he runs into a contradiction. It has been proven that plants also have interests: their roots grow deeper if necessary to absorb water or their stems grow towards the light. Studies on plant species demonstrate that they alert other plants so that they can prepare themselves for a parasite attack by releasing chemical substances. If we plant seeds of the same species, their roots do not compete with each other, but it we plant seeds of different species, they do. Some authors have even gone so far as to talk of plant intelligence [165] Should we give moral consideration to plants because of this?

There are people who think we should. A Swiss association has published documents claiming that plants have dignity and also deserve moral consideration and that, among other things, they should not be owned as property [166].

To conclude and to once again demonstrate the contradictions and arbitrary positions that Singer's vision can lead to if the capacity to feel pain is the north star that defines membership or not of the moral community, we could argue that worms are part of it since they are able to learn how to avoid unpleasant sensations [167]. Even some unicellular organisms, such as paramecia, would belong to this moral community, as rigorous studies have demonstrated they also avoid unpleasant sensations by assimilating and avoiding negative stimuli. What's more, their learning is accelerated if they are exposed to the same stimuli repeatedly. This opens up the possibility that they have memory, albeit not a synaptic memory but one mediated by organic molecules [168].

Therefore, the interest of these organisms, which are capable of experiencing unpleasant sensations (since they avoid them), in not having such sensations should have the same moral consideration as our desire not to experience negative sensations. This could lead us to absurd situations, such as protecting the life of parasites or bacteria.

Giving moral consideration or not to other living beings is arbitrary since these beings don't demand or even understand it. This arbitrary nature can lead us to paradoxical, undesirable and even dangerous, profoundly unethical situations.

In 2017, the Government of Saudi Arabia granted full citizenship to Sophia. Every country in the world naturalises foreign citizens through administrative processes. Nothing noteworthy then, except for the fact that Sophia is not a woman, she is not even a human. Sophia is a robot [169].

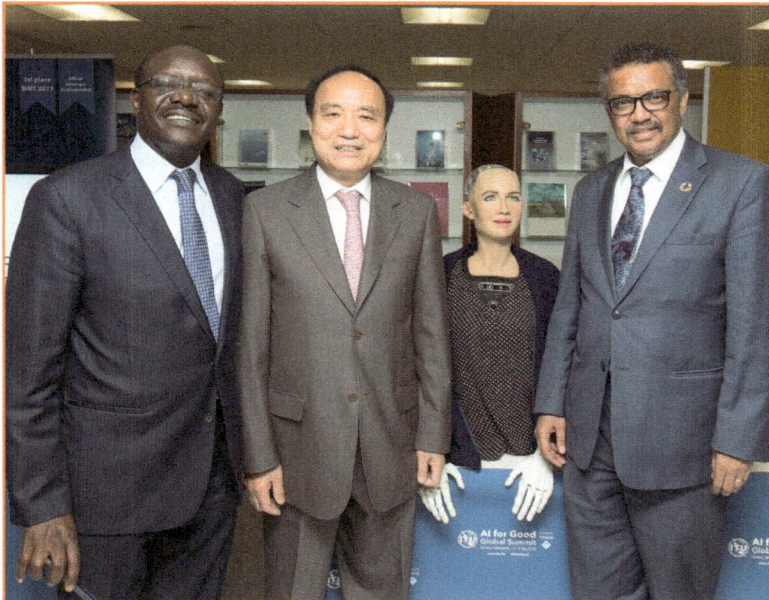

The robot citizen Sophia accompanied by various directors of international organisations.

That a humanoid is granted such a right is disconcerting, even more so in a country where the rights and liberties granted to women are particularly limited.

Should we grant rights to robots if they start to have the capacity to suffer or if they become unique, different from all the others, with their own incipient personality, as is starting to be the case?

More proof that humanisation, in this case of an object, is a pathway to the dehumanisation of people.

Do robots deserve to have rights? After all, Sophia is capable of holding a simple conversation with someone. She modulates her voice depending on how she perceives the mood of the person talking to her and, over time, learns to adapt her behaviour depending on what she has heard previously. Therefore, it's not a robot than can be immediately replaced with another. Evidently, she doesn't feel pain nor does she have self-awareness but we can't really know how a shrimp experiences pain or what level of consciousness a sea cucumber has either.

And there's already an association for the prevention of cruelty to robots [170] and in academia some voices are already asking for this recognition, although in a more limited form compared to the recognition humans enjoy [171].

HitchBOT was a robot created to hitch-hike. In tests conducted with it in Canada and Europe, it managed to get to its destination. It was programmed to maintain a simple conversation and provide company to the drivers who gave it a lift. In what turned out to be its last trip from the east coast of the USA to California, its journey came to an abrupt end in Philadelphia, where it was found decapitated and completely destroyed. It was not lucky enough to be protected by legislation [172]. Is this a vandalism or a crime? If HitchBOT or any other robot has rights similar to those of citizens, should the person who attacked it be charged with a criminal offence and punished in a way that goes beyond fines for the material value of the robot?

Once the door to the moral community has been opened to animals, why stop at animals? Why not extend it to plants and some robots?

In fact, there are attempts to make robots behave in a more inclusive and ethical way [173] and a Google engineer was recently sacked because he claimed he couldn't tell whether he was talking to a human or an algorithm (LaMDA) he was working on. He also claimed that LaMDA expressed its fear of being disconnected [174]. Are we on the verge of silicon consciousness competing with our own? Will algorithms deserve rights or can we switch them off?

The reader might have a different view but I think there are more than enough arguments to believe that giving rights to robots or to mice and refusing to give them to some people is profoundly unjust, immoral and heinous.

We shouldn't forget that all animals defend themselves and give priority to their own species. The instinct of self-preservation, like that of reproduction, is intimately linked to our nature, to our biology. So why shouldn't we act in the same way and give priority to our fellow humans, to our species? What reasoning should lead us to consider animals or robots as equals and put them on the same social, legal or moral plane as ourselves?

Singer based his belief on the capacity of a living creature to feel pain or pleasure. Let us pause for a moment and consider this point. Should pain be the benchmark for the moral consideration of an animal?

Pain as a moral reference or why pain is an opinion

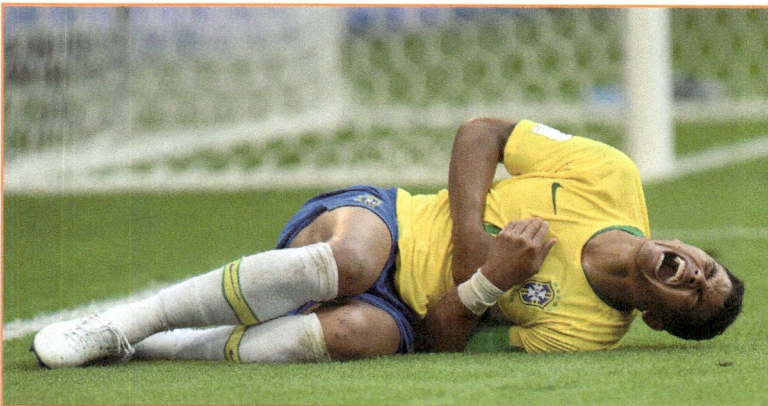

Pain is a subjective sensation and, therefore, varies depending on the person and the context.

We owe the memorable phrase "pain is an opinion" to the Indian-American neurologist V. S. Ramachandran, who obtained his doctorate at Cambridge and is considered a global authority of the study of phantom limbs, synaesthesia and other key aspects of how the nervous system functions. In one of his books Ramachandran explains:

> "Pain is an opinion on the organism's state of health rather than a mere reflexive response to an injury. There is no direct hotline from pain receptors to 'pain centres' in the brain. There is so much interaction between different brain centres, like those concerned with vision and touch, that even the mere visual appearance of an opening fist can actually feed all the way back into the patient's motor and touch pathways, allowing him to feel the fist opening, thereby killing an illusory pain in a non-existent hand". [175]

The text has its origins in an experiment he conducted on patients who felt significant pain in limbs that had been amputated. This is known as phantom limb syndrome [176]. Ramachandran designed a box with mirrors so that the patient would see the hand that they hadn't lost in the place where the amputated hand would have been. The visualisation of this mirror image of the healthy hand in the place of the amputated hand completely eliminated the pain and phantom limb syndrome [177].

We have seen the fundamental importance that the capacity to suffer, to feel pain has for Singer and how it leads him to include animals, at least up to crustaceans (from molluscs onwards he has some doubts), in the sphere of the moral community.

Now, if pain is the guide we are using to determine who belongs or does not belong to this community, we have to define very clearly what pain is, how it manifests and how it is measured. Otherwise we'll fall into arbitrariness and even contradictions in how we classify a being moral or non-moral.

The International Association for the Study of Pain [178] defines it as "an unpleasant sensory and emotional experience associated with ... actual or potential tissue damage" [179]. We perceive the sensation of physical pain through receptors known as nociceptors, which are distributed throughout the body.

These pain receptors are present in all vertebrates, as well as in insects, worms, leeches, molluscs and slugs [180].

However, the capacity to feel unpleasant sensations via nociceptors and pain are not the same thing.

Pain is a subjective experience, we have all seen how the same injury, for example a scratch on the knee, can trigger an explosive outburst of pain from a child yet pass totally unnoticed in an adult.

There are numerous reports in which soldiers and injured people say they did not feel any pain despite having very serious injuries [181].

We have already seen how animals have the same pain receptors as humans, although the African mole-rat is an interesting exception to this rule. This species of rodent doesn't feel pain from acid or other irritants [182]. Should it therefore be excluded from the moral community claimed by some animal rights philosophers?

Clearly, both human and animal suffering is not limited to the experience of physical pain. Mood and psychological factors, such as stress, can cause profound suffering even without physical pain being involved. However, if the experience of pain has a strong subjective component, suffering is even more difficult to quantify.

Both human and animal suffering is not limited to the experience of physical pain. Mood and psychological factors, such as stress, can cause profound suffering.

In a subway train carriage full of passengers first thing in the morning, everyone is crammed together, their physical environment in terms of temperature, humidity, proximity to one other, etc., is the same. However, in this same carriage, there are happy people, depressed people, people in pain, worried people and hopeful people. The level of happiness or sadness they are feeling varies greatly depending on thousands of factors.

This is relevant because it is essential to separate moral consideration from such subjective and variable elements like pain and suffering. We have already seen examples of people and animals who are immune to pain: should they be outside the moral community? Where do we draw the line between sentient and non-sentient beings and what determines whether they are sentient or not? Nociceptors? The mental capacity to suffer? An oyster or an eel can feel pain, but can they also suffer?

Even the presence of nociceptors is not synonymous with feeling pain – or at least not to the same extent that we humans do. In fact, insects' behaviour casts doubt on this correlation since grasshoppers and crickets with very serious injuries continue to use the injured limb as if nothing had happened. There are even insects that will continue to feed while being eaten by a bigger insect. We also have the case of male mantids, which will continue to mate even as they are being eaten by their partners [183].

Fish, although they have pain receptors, do not show pain in the same way as other vertebrates immediately after a surgical intervention [184].

This all demonstrates that using suffering and pain as a basis and guide to determine who is or isn't within the moral community – as some utilitarians want to do – is far more arbitrary than limiting that community to humans.

It is obvious that, however subjective painful experiences or what we define as suffering may be, these negative sensations must be minimised or eliminated in domesticated animals. Always. Certainly suffering, in certain circumstances, may be unavoidable, or the lesser of two evils, but it is profoundly immoral to provoke it in a sentient being without a very good reason.

Are human beings just another animal?

Another idea that we find more and more in anti-speciesist arguments in particular – but also in the scientific field in general – is the idea that the human beings should be considered as just another animal. Our physiology, neurology and behaviour are ultimately, many argue, only slightly different from those of most animals. After all, our genetic code is practically identical to that of a chimpanzee and we share 50% of our genes with *drosophila*, also known as fruit flies. Given all of the above, we might ask why, since we are so closely related to our animal cousins, we should establish significant differences with regard to the moral treatment that some receive compared to others. In fact, the difference between the characteristics that make us human and those that animals have – or at least a lot of them – would just be one of degree and not of nature [185].

It seems that, more or less implicitly, it is important for animal rights activists, and seemingly some scientists as well, to equate us to animals and vice versa. They claim we should reject the anthropocentric view of the natural world and adopt a more zoocentric perspective. Given that the observed differences between humans and animals are of degree and not of nature, the way some animals use tools can be equated to the way we do. The chimpanzee that uses a stone to crack a nut would be doing the same as a team of engineers capable of putting a satellite in orbit. The difference would merely be one of degree, the animal-human boundary would be arbitrary [186].

Using suffering and pain as a basis and guide to determine who is or isn't within the moral community – as some utilitarians want to do – is far more arbitrary than limiting that community to humans.

This approach is striking since if, as Regan argues, animals have value in themselves or, as Singer does, only the capacity to suffer is relevant with regard to the right to belong to the moral community, it should be irrelevant how close or otherwise animals are behaviourally or genetically to people. Nevertheless, it seems that anthropocentrism has not been completely rejected in the animal rights world [187], because these groups are obsessed with making humans more animal and animals more human (their own jargon demonstrates this with their insistence on calling animals non-human animals or non-human persons).

This understanding ignores the fact that humans are the only living beings that have made themselves a moral species and, therefore, we judge our fellow humans and our own behaviour as good or bad, humane or inhumane, as right or wrong, as moral or immoral. If a human being is just another species, why should we behave differently to other species. After all, all species favour their own species, in other words they are speciesist. But if, on the other hand, human beings, by virtue of the fact that they are moral, must give moral consideration or status to other species, then in that case, they are already considered *de facto* different from other animals and implicitly superior in terms of judgement and intellectual capacity.

The natural sciences are able to explain very well how much animal there is in humans (indeed, there is no doubt that we are anatomically and physiologically animals), but not what transcends our animality and makes us people. Genetics, biochemistry and histology doesn't help us understand this aspect. We need to look at social sciences. Linguistics, politics, psychology and sociology explain – or at least try to – human beings, what it is that we have and that ultimately differentiates us from all other known species [188].

It is this idea, finding what distinguishes us from animals, that has occupied and, in a certain way, defined the *raison d'être* of philosophy since its very beginnings.

The history of this discipline provides us with different definitions and descriptions of what it is that makes us truly human: intelligence, self-awareness and the capacity to be free.

The time has come to consider how palaeontologists determine whether the fossil remains that they find of our humanoid ancestors belong to a human being or to an earlier species that still lacked the specific features that distinguish us. In addition to the morphological aspects that demonstrate the presence of linguistic ability – frontoparietal cranial development as well as the unique morphology of humans' middle ear ossicles – we have cultural findings such as the remains of stone and wood tools, the use and control of fire, the creation of artistic works and the presence of funeral rituals [189] [190]. Our way of dealing with death is a key aspect that explains the difference between humans and animals: a chimpanzee mother may carry her dead offspring for weeks, but once she abandons the body she cuts all ties with it. For humans, in contrast, the link to the dead never disappears. We build cemeteries for them, we honour their memory, they continue to be part of our lives [191].

> If human beings, by virtue of the fact that they are moral, must give moral consideration or status to other species, they are already considered *de facto* different from other animals and implicitly superior in terms of judgement and intellectual capacity.

All of this is unique and differentiates human beings (*Homo sapiens* from Neanderthals [192]) and distinguishes us from all other past and present apes. Furthermore, it's also a difference in nature compared to the rest of the animal kingdom. And while it's true that some animals use tools, they do so individually not in teams. And this is another of the chasms that separate us as species.

Argument by analogy

Authors as reputable as the British philosopher Hume [193] and Darwin himself [194] were firm believers in what we call today "argument by analogy", in other words that the similarity between a human behaviour and an animal behaviour has its roots in the similar mental states of the species. As a logical consequence, this view considers the differences between an ape and a human to be differences of degree rather than the result of different natures.

Is this hypothesis correct? We have already seen clear differences in this regard, but we can add some experiments investigating the issue conducted with chimpanzees [195]. Primates follow the gaze of their human interlocutor just as an 18 month old child would. There is no doubt that this a characteristic similar to one that humans have and one that the majority of species don't have. Does this mean that chimpanzees' gaze and our gaze serve the same function, that it should be interpreted in the same way in the two species?

For humans the link to the dead never disappears. We build cemeteries for them, we honour their memory, they continue to be part of our lives.

To answer this question, the chimpanzees were offered a treat in an experiment. In one case, one of the trainers had a bucket over their head so that the ape could not see the trainer's eyes. The other trainer did not cover their face. The chimpanzees did not distinguish between the two and asked for their treat both from the trainer who could see them and the trainer who couldn't. A similar experiment was performed with a trainer with their back turned and another with their back turned but their head turned to look at the animal. The response was the same. Unlike two year old children, who know who is looking at them and, therefore, who they should ask for their treat, the chimpanzees are not sensitive to gazes for this purpose [196].

In another experiment, a trainer fixed their gaze on one of two moulds under which he had hidden a treat. Three-year-old children picked the right mould every time and went for the mould the trainer was looking at. However, if the trainer did not look at either mould, they picked the right mould 50% of the time. In contrast, the chimpanzees only picked the right mould half the time in both cases. This confirms that, despite their excellent capacity to follow a gaze, chimpanzees don't realise how the gaze is related to subjective states of attention.

Unlike young humans, monkeys are not able to understand what it means when their trainer points to the right mould with their finger either.

> Assuming that a chimpanzee's and a human's gesture or gaze serve the same purpose, are used for the same thing or mean the same is completely wrong; there is a chasm between the intellectual and cognitive ability of a two-year-old child and an adult chimpanzee.

All of the above demonstrates that assuming that a chimpanzee's and a human's gesture or gaze serve the same purpose, are used for the same thing or mean the same is completely wrong and that there is indeed a chasm between the intellectual and cognitive ability of a two-year-old child and an adult chimpanzee. It is not simply a difference of degree. It is not that we do the same just with some differences. The simple fact is that, in many cases, we're not doing the same.

There is a whole range of literature that supports this idea. What the majority think explains certain simian behaviour – our supposed cognitive and psychological similarity – in fact has a very different explanation when tested scientifically.

As Michael Tomasello – professor of psychology and neurosciences at Duke University and co-director of the evolutionary anthropology department at the Max Planck Institute – explains, one thing that clearly distinguishes us from other species is our ability to cooperate. Cooperation that takes place between human beings who share a particular moment in time, as well as with those who preceded us.

Cooperating was key to our survival as a species and we encourage our children to do it, as they are more readily accepted in the community if they act in this way. We know what other people expect from us and we behave according to their expectations. As a result, children cheat less in a game if they are being observed by a third person compared to when they think no one will notice. In contrast, chimpanzees behave in the same way in both contexts [197].

Great apes follow the movements of another ape or person but what they're actually following is the movement of the head, not of the eyes. In fact, humans have a white sclera that allows us to see where the pupils are being directed when they focus on an object. Nine-month-old babies follow the head, babies over that age follow the eyes [198].

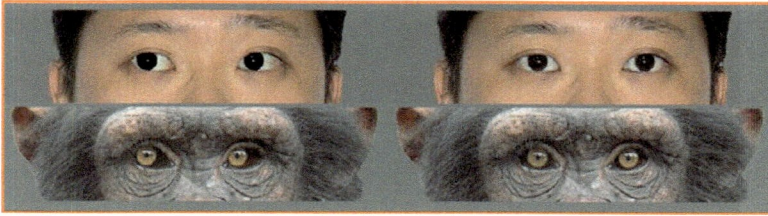

Human, and only human consciousness allows us to know what others are thinking and to anticipate their future reactions in certain situations, which results in significant competitive advantages [199].

This acting on behalf of others, in an altruistic way, anticipating the needs of others, is described very well by Tomasello [200] when he explains how twelve-month-old children indicate to an adult where to find an object that was put in one place by that adult and moved by another. Chimpanzees are incapable of doing the same. Nor do they understand what it means when someone points specifically to one of two boxes to indicate it contains food; they don't understand that someone wants to help them altruistically. Their communication is imperative: come, go, take, give to me. Not co-operative.

Another aspect explained by the same author is that an ape understands perfectly well when someone uses a hammer to crack a nut, but the same gesture in the absence of a tool or nut leaves them completely perplexed. They are unable to infer the gesture with the object if the object is not there.

This small selection of examples – there are many more – shows us that the difference between our psyche and evolution, not just as individuals but as a community, results in insuperable differences between us and the animals closest to us in the evolutionary chain.

We still don't know exactly what caused these differences, but if they were not enough in themselves, what we can class as evidence is that there are certain types of neurons that are only present in humans. These neurons are stimulated by the image of a specific person or simply the name of this person written on a piece of paper. These neurons are known as Jennifer Aniston neurons because their existence was first proven when the image of the American actress was used in experiments on epileptic patients. The fact that a concept – a name written down – stimulates a cell is unheard of in the animal kingdom, except in people.

The fact that a concept – a name written down – stimulates a cell is unheard of in the animal kingdom, except in people.

We are not capable of remembering everything that happens to us but we can memorise the concept, the general idea of a book, conference or a walk on the beach. To date, this capacity for synthesis and storing concepts has only been demonstrated in human beings [201].

In this eagerness to equate, to create a blank slate eliminating the difference between the animal and the human, some anti-speciesist authors don't just demand that animals should have rights, they even go so far as to claim that they should have access to certain forms of citizenship [202].

It is worth dwelling on this point, first of all, to emphasise the obvious: the concept of rights is completely alien to animals.

Declaring that all animals have an inalienable right to life, as some animal rights treatises claim [61], would condemn them all (or a large majority) to death since wolves have to eat deer to survive, and without wolves the deer population would multiply steadily until it reached a level that made its own ecosystem unsustainable. This has been shown by the need to reintroduce wolves into Yellowstone National Park [203] and the enormous environmental challenge presented by the banning of hunting in Cabañeros National Park in Castile-La Mancha, Spain. This ban led to an exponential increase in the deer and boar populations and required urgent measures to be taken to control the ungulate populations in the area [204].

Therefore, it's not a question of guaranteeing animals rights; to be the subject of rights you have to know what to do with them and know how to enforce them [205]. Understanding the concept of rights, which animals certainly do not, is vital in order to defend them. And while a mentally handicapped person may not understand them either, their fellow humans do, as we have seen previously.

As Adela Cortina [206] states "rights are demands for dignity, not resources or instruments from which utility is extracted". Therefore, it's not a question of giving animals rights but of imposing human obligations towards them. This is desirable and is already provided for in the more advanced legal systems of the world.

If someone harms a dog, the dog cannot claim their right not to be harmed. The dog's owner could complain and they might be compensated, but this wouldn't change anything for the dog in question.

Furthermore, having an obligation towards someone does not imply that this person acquires a right. To elaborate on this idea, we'll use the example given by the British legal philosopher H. L. A. Hart, who argued as follows [207]: "X promises Y, in return for some favour, that he will look after Y's aged mother in his absence. It would be person Y who possesses the right. X has an obligation to Y, therefore it is Y who possesses a right. Certainly, Y's mother is a person to whom X has acquired an obligation and Y could make a complaint against X if he doesn't fulfil his promise but there is no right to care for Y's mother". Having an obligation towards someone does not imply that this person has a right. The case of animals and babies is the same. Obligations towards them do not automatically transform into rights.

What is important for animals is that they are legally protected and that anyone who harms them is punished, not by the animals but by human society.

I fully agree with Singer and Regan that we should avoid causing pain to animals, but there are many reasons, which I have set out above, that, in my opinion, disqualify their arguments concerning giving equal moral consideration to humans and animals and, therefore, rights to the latter.

This point is key because giving rights to animals who don't know what they mean would be largely meaningless. What is important for animals is that they are legally protected and that anyone who harms them is punished, not by the animals but by human society.

This is the stumbling point of the argument set out by the authors of the Great Ape Project (GAP). They advocate that great apes should be legally granted human rights.

However, we also have to point out that genetic proximity (the fact that chimpanzees specifically and humans share 98% of our DNA) does not make us identical. Secondly, the GAP puts three species of apes (gorillas, chimpanzees and orangutans) in the same position, even though their genetic proximity to humans is very different, as are their cognitive abilities.

Nevertheless, beyond counting genes or chromosomes (in the end, DNA is made up of 4 bases A, G, C and T, so any DNA we design from these bases will share a certain percentage with our own), what must be made clear is that genetics, however important its findings may be, does not explain the entirety of a being or a community.

The fact that we share 50% of our genes with fruit flies does not mean we are half fly or that they are half human.

Let's look at the example of an eagle. This marvellous animal can fly, hunt, has extraordinary eyesight and an internal skeleton. Let's now consider an eagle's egg: it can't fly, it can't hunt, it can't see and its protective system is an exterior one – the eggshell. However, genetically the egg and the eagle are identical. A neuron and an intestinal epithelial cell are also genetically identical. The former transmits nervous impulses and is star-shaped, while the latter secretes mucus and absorbs nutrients. What differentiates them is how each gene is expressed at any given moment.

In the same way, if an ape or a person behave, feed themselves and reproduce differently, if they occupy different biological niches and are easy to distinguish anatomically, why should all these differences be sacrificed on the altar of a supposed genetic proximity? The fact that we share 50% of our genes with fruit flies does not mean we are half fly or that they are half human [208].

The quantitatively minor chromosomal difference manifests itself in qualitatively huge differences.

Human beings possess language, the ability to give guttural sounds an arbitrary meaning that allows us to share past, present and future experiences; language allows us to narrate imaginary events, desires, invent new worlds, explain how a nuclear reactor works or pray to a god. And it is perfectly developed in every human society on earth. No animal, however evolved it is or genetically close it is, has anything similar because, to put it simply, they are not human.

Guaranteeing human rights to non-humans on the basis of their genetics is also socially dangerous because it could open the door to claiming different rights for people with chromosomal differences. Only sovereign states can grant citizenship and, with it, rights. Assigning these rights on the basis of the number of chromosomes and genetics would take us back to previous eras when humans were also catalogued on the basis of a supposed racial profile based on hereditary characteristics. Nothing good came from those ideologies.

Of course, apes – like many other animals – should be protected and their ecosystems preserved. I don't think anyone disagrees with that. Unfortunately, respect for human rights *for humans* is not always the norm in those regions. Respect for the environment, and thus for animals, improves very significantly as a society's quality of life improves [209]. It is, therefore, imperative to respect the duties we have towards apes and their preservation by upholding the rights and welfare of the people who share their land with them.

As Jonathan Marks, an anthropologist at the University of North Carolina, explains: "a suffering chimpanzee may be genetically 98% human but a suffering person is 100% human" [208].

Therefore, in my opinion it is profoundly immoral to grant equal rights to animals, to include them in the moral collective or, in other words, to leave out of this collective people who, for various reasons, have lost or simply do not possess the abilities that distinguish us as humans, namely the ability to think and imagine the future, the abstraction that allows us to attribute meaning to arbitrary sounds, respect for the dead, and respect for their last wishes to name but a few examples. Losing these abilities doesn't stop them from being fathers, mothers, friends or citizens fully worthy of respect and protection.

They are human, they intrinsically possess humanity and they don't stop being human just because their capacities are not perfectively active.

Ortega y Gasset's dictum is revealing in this context: "Humankind has no nature, only history" [210]. Indeed, people's lives take place in a given historical context. Life is not the same for a woman born in Europe in the 2000s as it would have been for a woman born on the same continent in the 19th century. Furthermore, as individuals we mould our own existence, we change it, we can alter it (we haven't stopped doing this since the start of history). Thus, the Spanish philosopher claimed: "As it is not bound to a fixed and immutable constant – to a "nature" – it is free to be, or at least try to be, whatever it wants. That is why man is free and … not by coincidence".

> **Not all lives have the same possibilities and the same potential. Therefore, placing them on the same level does not give a higher value to the lives of animals – which remain removed from our debates – but lowers the value we give to humans. And that, in my opinion, is immoral.**

In contrast, animals have no history. No matter what era lions live or lived in, life is pretty much the same for all lions, regardless of when and where they were born: they hunted, they reproduced, they fought to lead their pride, and they died. Therefore, it is unthinkable that parallels can be drawn between the value of a human and an animal life or that animals can be described as non-human persons, attempting to group animality and humanity as one. By trying to elevate the former, they degrade the latter.

Not all lives have the same possibilities and the same potential. Therefore, placing them on the same level does not give a higher value to the lives of animals – which remain removed from our debates – but lowers the value we give to humans. And that, in my opinion, is immoral. It is not so much the diet a person chooses – each to their own – but the root causes of such behaviour that lead me to conclude that a person who doesn't eat animal products because they equate animal and human lives is immoral and is not on a higher ethical plane, but quite the opposite. There are not human and non-human persons. There are animals and people. That doesn't mean we love or respect animals any less, but rather that we dignify human beings.

The point is that the proponents of these theories use science as a smokescreen, as a cover for a goal that is not limited to protecting apes but is, in fact, to eliminate all animal husbandry, all animal experimentation and even, in the most extreme cases, all ownership of animals – including domestic cats and dogs. And the misrepresentation of science can, in some cases, act as an alibi for this purpose. However, as soon as a paper demonstrates the falsity of some of the theories used by animal rights activists, it is quickly buried or, failing that, denigrated. In contrast, any study – or interpretation of a study – that supports their position is amplified on websites and social networks where, admittedly, these associations move with manifest skill.

Nevertheless, it remains the case that animals, including the most evolved, occupy a different sphere to humans. This is not to take value away from animals nor to reduce one iota our obligation to preserve their ecosystems. On the contrary. Let us love them, admire them, protect them for what they are, not for what some would like them to be.

3. THE CONSEQUENCES OF AN ANTI-SPECIESIST WORLD

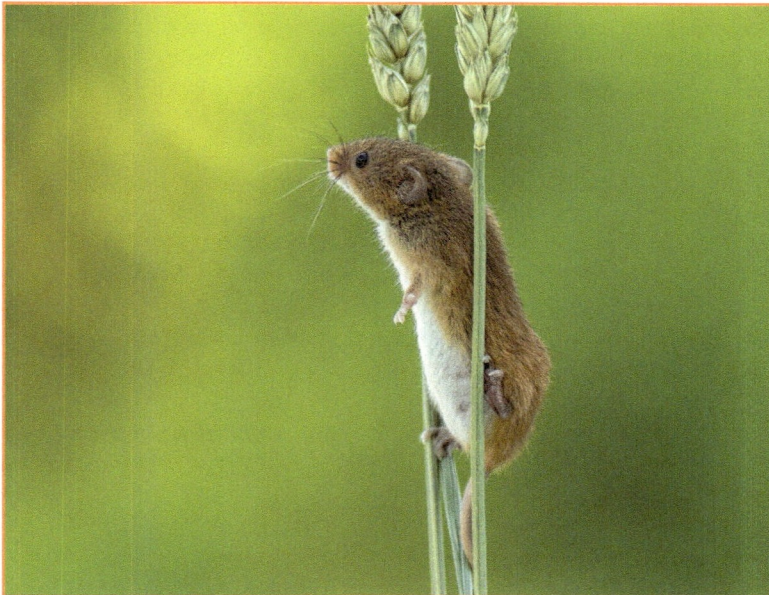

We have responded in detail to the philosophy of Tom Regan and we have explained why we can and should make a radical and profound distinction between animals and disabled human beings. We have seen why membership of the category of sentient beings should not necessarily be the characteristic that allows animals to be elevated to the category of moral beings as Peter Singer claims.

So, let's now ask the following question from a utilitarian perspective: is being vegan moral? At first glance, it would seem that it is. The immense majority of vegans adopt the philosophy with good intentions and I would go so far as to claim that a lot of omnivores, although they prefer not to change diet, view reducing the consumption of meat and the rise of the vegetarian diet favourably.

Nevertheless, let's look in depth at what a vegan world would really look like. If the tenets of this philosophy were imposed, we would have a society without the consumption of meat, milk, honey, eggs or wool; without animals for experimentation; without the strength that animals provide to pull heavy loads or a plough; without their products in the pharmacopoeia; without control of invasive species; without animals for pet food - in fact without dogs and cats because they need meat to live and grow - without the possibility of getting rid of rodents or insects when they become a threat to crops or grain stores or grain stores, when they parasitise us directly, or when they could be carrying diseases that affect us or other animals.

The vegan approach would have all these limitations because, if animals deserve consideration in their own right, as Regan claims, they should be respected in the same way as we respect people. And if their capacity to suffer makes them moral beings as Singer claims, they also deserve the same consideration as us and, therefore, all the uses of animals mentioned above would be explicitly banned.

However, let's analyse in more detail the consequences of such bans to see if the resulting vegan world would transform humanity for the better or not.

From this perspective, can we consider as moral to put human and animal life at the same level? What would happen, hypothetically, if we all became anti-speciesists overnight?

Let's see:

In such a scenario, every animal on every farm all over the world would stop having any commercial value as no one would consume their products. Of course, we would be concerned for their welfare – that's why we've all become vegans, to not consume any of their products – so we can't slaughter them. Nor can we free them – except for a few exceptions – because the vast majority wouldn't be able to survive outside the farm (they lost their ability to survive in the wild when they were domesticated) or because, if they could survive, they might be a threat to native wildlife (as would be the case for the American mink or salmon, which would become a danger to local species if released). Therefore, the most humane thing to do would be to keep them on the farm until they die of natural causes. However, this alternative isn't very ethical either since someone would have to look after them and the farmers – as they don't have any financial incentive – would not be able to assume the cost of food, veterinary care, air conditioning, water, electricity or gas, repairs, pest control (which would be another contradiction), medicines, and other supplies that are vital for keeping the livestock in optimal condition. But let's not forget that, according to the majority of vegans, conditions on farms are dreadful, so these animals would be prolonging this agony until their natural demise – several years in the majority of cases. Furthermore, the animals wouldn't have their freedom to reproduce limited since, if they deserve the same moral consideration as people, we shouldn't castrate them or limit their ability to procreate. Therefore, in all likelihood, the problem of overcrowding, poor care, high mortality and the risk of infections would increase exponentially and would potentially drag on forever.

There would also be other paradoxes we would find hard to reconcile: we wouldn't be able to perform rat or pest control in the buildings the animals are housed in. There is no doubt this would contribute to the spread of diseases and lower the animals' state of welfare because the rodents and parasites take food, as well as causing stress, injury and illness in the animals.

And we have to find a balance between the different interests.

The animals wouldn't see their living conditions improve nor would we be able to free them. Maintaining them would, therefore, require altruistic donors or the state to assume the costs of their upkeep. These are resources that, if they could be found, would be taken away from other productive actions or from other collectives that potentially need them more.

No, it definitely wouldn't be a better world. On the other hand, all perishable products of animal origin – milk, eggs, meat, fish – would have to be destroyed because no one would consume them, and leaving them to rot would have an enormous environmental impact and keeping them frozen would be hugely expensive and pointless given they wouldn't be used at any point in the future. Even non-perishable animal products, such as wool and leather, that haven't yet been sold would be destroyed or warehoused *sine die* since there wouldn't be any demand for them in a new strict vegan world.

The animals transform what we can't, vegetable remains and animals that don't have any value to us into protein of high biological value.

Some will claim – Singer himself does so – that the change would have to be a gradual one because education and raising awareness to encourage the adoption of a vegan diet requires time and, ultimately, the transition would have to be phased in. However, this approach does not prevent the problem. At some point, farms will stop being profitable and, at that point, the process described above would be triggered.

The negative effects of a vegan world don't stop there. A strict vegan diet, giving up food of animal origin, is difficult to implement. Not impossible, but difficult for sure. We'll dedicate a full chapter to this subject.

In a scenario like the one described: how would we feed millions of people for whom livestock is the only source of protein and other basic nutrients in their diet? The animals transform what we can't; for example, vegetable remains that don't have any value to us into protein of high biological value. In fact, livestock farming was born to use animals as recyclers of what we couldn't digest but animals could: fruit peel, worm-eaten tubers, their own faeces, the remains of game such as skins, feathers or guts, eggshells, shellfish shells, and much much more. Livestock converts all this into meat or milk or wool that will then be very useful for the community. Today livestock continues to play this recycler function, as we will describe later on. What response would anti-speciesism give to these billions of people?

But let's continue with the consequences of a vegan world. What would we do in the event that barns or the harvests themselves are invaded by insects or rodents? If all animals always have the right to life under all circumstances, we'll have to accept that we can't implement pest control measures in fields and silos or at food companies. Bear in mind that rodents destroy a very substantial proportion of the world's cereal crops, as well as other crops. In Asia, on a yearly basis, these species consume an amount of grain that could feed 200 million people [211]. In Tanzania, they eat between 5–15% of the harvest each year, which is a quantity equivalent to the amount eaten by 2 million of its inhabitants. The damage done to the grain once it is in the silos is no less significant. Here, the animals can destroy more than 10% of the grain stored [212]. Nor are developed countries immune to rodents and fruit-eating birds. The damage they do to agriculture in California, to give just one example, is also significant [213].

That's without taking into account the risks to health that rats represent. Their faeces and mere presence as carriers of viruses and bacteria can lead to the transmission of more than 50 diseases to humans and livestock. Let's imagine, therefore, a world in which rats and mice have inalienable rights equivalent to those of humans, as Regan extolled and as many vegan associations continue to extol, and roam wild and unchecked. That's not to mention the insects, snails, slugs and other invertebrates that compete with us for the fruits in the fields. To give one example, since the start of 2021, Kenya has been suffering a locust plague, with 80 million insects per square kilometre. Every day this plague eats a quantity equivalent to the amount needed to feed 35,000 people [214]. I don't know if animal rights activists believe these arthropods have intrinsic value and that we should, therefore, respect their lives but given the consideration they give to bees [215], the response would be yes since I don't think there is a big difference in capabilities, perception of reality and capacity to feel between grasshoppers and honeybees.

> **Livestock farming was born to use animals as recyclers of what we couldn't digest but animals could: fruit peel, worm-eaten tubers, egg shells, shellfish shells… Livestock converts all this into meat or milk or wool that will then be very useful for the community.**

What can you say? What should we do when an animal parasitises us directly? How should we react if we ourselves or our pets are attacked by fleas, mites or mosquitoes? Can we defend ourselves or should we risk suffering serious infections? How can we coexist with and respect a mite that has made a home for itself in our groin? After all, insects and arachnids have some very advanced perceptions, most probably not very different from the bees that animal rights associations venerate.

Let's imagine a world in which rats and mice have inalienable rights equivalent to those of humans and roam wild and unchecked.

And what about worms in our intestine, liver or even eyes. Should they also be part of the moral community? Even though, in principle, the mental activity and sentience of worms is highly questionable, we shouldn't forget that some human beings may have their mental capacities diminished to such an extent that we could draw comparisons between them and some worms. Do they therefore deserve the same moral consideration as animal rights philosophers claim?

If animals cannot be used as instruments to achieve our aims, we shouldn't use them for transport or to carry loads either. In many regions of the third world, oxen that plough fields are still key to harvesting some crops from the soil. Without them, hunger – never too far away – would be inevitable [216]. What's more, the majority of working animals are neutered so they are easier to control and this practice would have to be abandoned with the resulting risks for farmers. Some islands have been able to legally ban motor vehicles from their territory (and replaced them with mules), for example Hydra in Greece or Mackinac Island in Lake Huron in the USA, but they would have to allow cars back in for transport. Land that is hard to access, such as coffee plantations in Guatemala where today 85% of the harvest is transported by horses, would have to be abandoned [216].

Some might think it's an exaggeration to claim that animal rights groups would oppose the use of working animals when their absence would have such nefarious consequences for a lot of communities. However, these associations are very vocal in their protests against the use of horse-drawn carriages in cities [217] [218]. Their protests against the use of horses to pull carriages, reported in the media in several countries, have resulted in the disappearance of these animals from some cities, for example Rome [219].

Pony rides, enjoyed by quite a few Parisian children, could have their days numbered if the demands of the animal rights party, which has seats on the city council, are met. In addition to a direct ban, these groups want to make it impossible in practice to use the horses, with draconian measures such as requiring them to rest one in every three days or to take maternity leave [220], which makes it almost impossible to make the activity financial viable.

I don't see how the life of a donkey in Ethiopia is much better than that of a horse in Chicago. Animal rights activists would almost certainly oppose both uses. The reader can draw their own conclusions.

It's curious to see how, wherever anti-speciesists manage to impose their beliefs, animals do not get better living conditions or quality of life, they simply disappear.

ANIMAL PHARMACOPOEIA

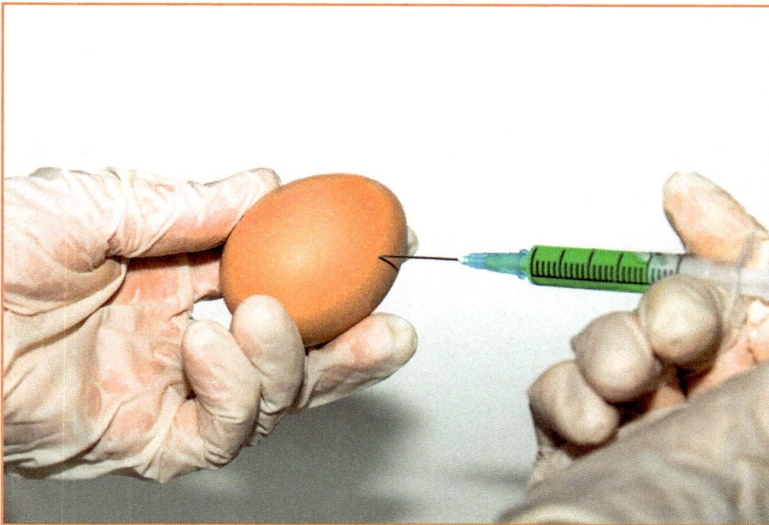

Obviously, if we can't slaughter animals, we will be obliged to go without some medications that we can only get from animals. After all, even though these medicines save the lives of millions of people every year, for the animal rights collective, this is all academic if it's at the expense of animal deaths. Heparin is perhaps the most paradigmatic case. This compound is an anticoagulant widely used in the treatment of circulatory disease such as thrombosis. It's on the WHO's list of essential medicines.

What should we do when an animal parasitises us directly? How should we react if we ourselves or our pets are attacked by fleas, mites or mosquitoes?

It is a natural compound found in some animal mucosa. Today, the drug is taken from the intestinal mucosa of pigs. To obtain the amount needed for treatments that could save the lives of around 100 million people, we need to collect the product from a total of 800 million pigs [221].

There are a lot of other treatments that have their origins in animal substances, examples include colloidal surfactants (protein-based liquid that coats the surface of the lungs), whose absence can cause newborn babies to asphyxiate. Pigs also provide the solution here. To continue with pigs, we should mention the pig heart valves implanted to treat a lot of heart diseases.

Lots of other species, for example cows, make numerous contributions to human health. Let's use a polygeline-based drug as an example. This drug is used to compensate or prevent circulatory failure caused by an absolute or relative plasma or blood volume deficit, as happens for example in cases of significant blood loss.

Polygeline is a bovine gelatin (extracted from bone) derivative composed of polypeptides that is prescribed for the aforementioned clinical cases and administered intravenously to rapidly restore plasma volume [222].

Birds also form part of the animal pharmacopoeia – how could they not? Thanks to them we have hyaluronic acid, a natural polysaccharide used to treat knee osteoarthritis and even, among high-performance athletes, used as a cure for sprained ankles. The synthesis of this product is complex and the principal source for the industry producing it is the crests of chickens and hens, which are very rich in this nutrient.

Staying with birds, there is no doubt that their most important contribution comes in the production of vaccines. These preventative medicines, which have possibly done the most to increase human life expectancy, are made up of microorganisms that, although dead or weakened, stimulate our defences without causing any harm to us. However, for viruses to reproduce, they need live cells. Embryonic chicken eggs are often used for this purpose. The developing embryo provides a source of rapidly reproducing cells that are an ideal growth medium for numerous viruses.

Despite the huge quantity of eggs – and other products of animal origin such as gelatin – used to make vaccines, the majority of vegans, fortunately, do not refuse them [223] [224].

Let's end this section, which could be a book in itself, with a final example: ursodeoxycholic acid. In the 1970s, this compound was discovered to have healing properties: it was capable of dissolving cholesterol gallstones, and alleviating other liver problems. In the 2000s, it was approved by the FDA and European Medicines Agency for these illnesses. Slightly later, towards 2015, a Chinese company that was manufacturing the product found a method for obtaining the active substance from chicken bile taken from remains at slaughterhouses. Today, this is the principal source of the drug [225].

I don't know how many lives would have been lost without the cures provided by animals but I have no doubts the number would be several hundred million every year. Would it be moral to stop producing these medicines?
The life of a human always has more value than that of an animal.

I don't know how many lives would have been lost without these cures provided by animals but I have no doubt that the number would be several hundred million every year. Would it be moral to stop producing these medicines? We have already seen why the life of a human always has more value than that of an animal, therefore I think we can conclude that the answer is no. Clearly not everyone agrees, although perhaps the majority of strict vegans are not aware of a lot of the ways that products of animal origin are used.

INVASIVE SPECIES

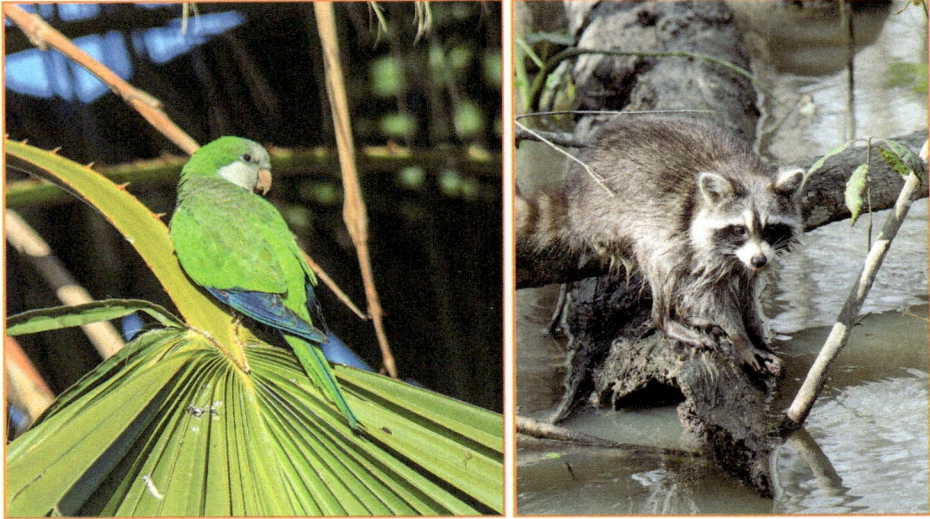

Another case where the right to respect the life of certain animals is arguable is the case of invasive species. According to the International Union for Conservation of Nature (IUCN), if a species is introduced outside of its current or historical natural range and it becomes problematic, then it must be considered an invasive species [226]. One of the solutions that this agency proposes in some cases is the eradication of the invasive species.

However, invasive species generally pose more of a threat to other animals than to humans, making it a morally easier choice, since we have to choose between one or the other. There are multiple examples and, in all of them, the impact of the foreign species on the local fauna is very negative. Examples include the Argentinian parrots in Spanish cities, the feral camels of Australia, the zebra mussel in the Great Lakes in North America, the lionfish in the Caribbean, the Asian python snakes adapted to the wetlands of the US state of Florida, the invasive California king snakes that have invaded some of the Canary Islands, and the tiger mosquito that has recently appeared in peninsula Spain. The American mink is perhaps the most paradigmatic case. This invasive species, which is now present practically throughout the northern half of peninsular Spain, has adapted well to the land to which it was introduced in 1950s as a result of escapes from fur farms [227]. Although it is not the main reason for their presence in our countryside, the contribution of animal rights groups to their expansion through entering mink farms and "liberating" them should not be underestimated [228] [229]. Of course, the damage it is doing to local fauna is incalculable: from the displacement of the native European mink through to putting at risk the mere existence of some local species not prepared for a new predator. For example, around 60% of heron chicks in La Nava lagoon in Palencia fell prey to the American mink [230]. Argentina is also suffering the same problem and some species of bird are particularly affected [231]. Invasive species are a global problem.

Furthermore, these "liberated" animals – or their offspring – are going to be hunted and ultimately slaughtered under local and international legislation that regulates the control of invasive species. As a result, the American mink has already been eliminated from the Hebrides in Scotland, and Spanish autonomous communities have programmes for trapping and eliminating the mustelid [232]. It is sad self-deception on the part of these "animal liberators", who contribute to the death of a significant part of the local fauna by releasing a few farm animals that will end up being hunted [233] [234] and possibly eradicated from a territory they should never have been released into.

THE PARTICULAR CASE
OF ANIMAL EXPERIMENTATION

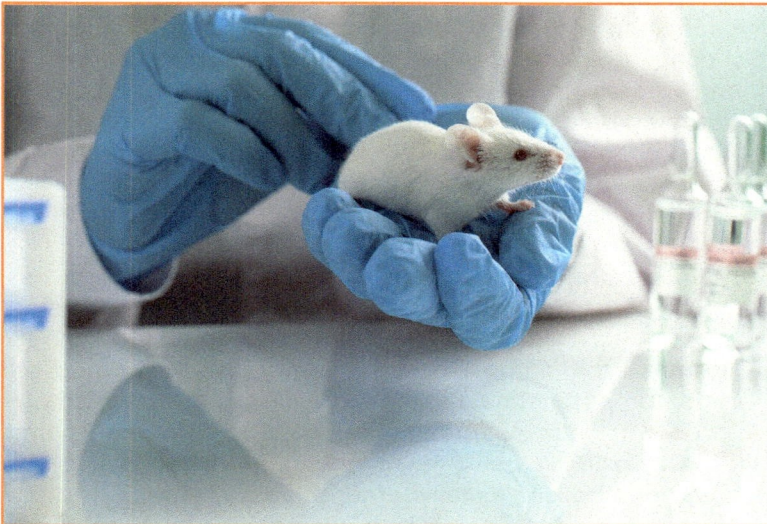

In 1622, the Milanese physician Gaspare Aselli described the vessels that made up the lymphatic system. To make this observation, he had performed a vivisection on a dog, which he fattened in order to make the lymph vessels more visible. The whole procedure was performed without anaesthesia, which did not exist at the time. The horror of the practice did not prevent its use. It was common in those times, especially in light of the Church's ban on dissecting human corpses [235]. Cartesian ideas claimed that animals did not feel pain [236] and that their howls were like the sound of a clock destroyed with a hammer, simple echoes of broken pieces. This idea was so dominant that another physician Olaus Rudbeck, still in the 17th century, cut up more than 400 animals (cats, wolves, cows and dogs amongst others) to continue investigating the lymphatic system [237].

Since the time of Ancient Greece, other doctors before them had used the same methods to learn more about the inside of the body and to try to find out how it worked. The suffering inflicted on thousands of animals was surely indescribable and unjustified, since the same knowledge could have been obtained by performing autopsies on corpses.

There is also no doubt that animals have always been used as a reference [238], a mirror in which we try to find our own anatomical and physiological self. Today, animal research continues to be vital for obtaining medicines that save millions of lives (human and animal). Of course, the legislation and control concerning these experiments is very strict. Avoiding suffering to animals is the foremost concern of the researchers, as it should be and, as we will see, despite what several animal rights groups claim [239]. If we want medical progress to continue, we can't give up experimentation. Why is the involvement of animals in research essential? For several reasons:

1 A lot of drugs that seem effective at an early stage have to be discarded after testing in animals. While this might seem to cast doubt on the benefit of such tests, it is in fact a sign of their importance. While a system of cultured cells or a computer simulation may give us clues as to how the drug will behave, nothing will give us as much information as a living being, with its multiple organs and complex metabolism, as to whether the drug is effective or not, whether it is toxic or not and, ultimately, whether it can be

tested on a limited basis in humans before being approved for marketing. Animal experimentation makes it possible to rule out a great many molecules because, thanks to guinea pigs, mice or monkeys, we already know that they will not provide a cure for the disease in question [240] [241].

2 Once the drug has passed these tests, we need to find out what the most effective dose is, what side effects can be expected when it's taken, whether or not it can be used in all age groups, whether or not it is risky for pregnant women, how it behaves when administered with other drugs or in patients with prior diseases. All these questions are answered thanks to animal testing.

Animal rights activists are completely obsessed with opposing this practice. They use several spurious reasons to try to demonstrate its limited value [242]. They even take advantage of the popularity of their arguments among some celebrities to get them to appear in videos, for example, the actress who played Sheldon Cooper's always dissatisfied girlfriend in The Big Bang Theory. Although she has a background in neuroscience in real life, she presents very weak arguments against animal testing [243]. However, this does not detract one iota from the power these advertising campaigns have to convince a population that is unaware of the causes and effects of animal research and the dire consequences its banning would have.

The reality is that, beyond the propaganda, without lab animals it would have been impossible to develop an anti-COVID-19 vaccine, to give a recent example of enormous social and medical importance [244] [245].

Less friendly than the campaigns featuring familiar actors are the threats, aggression and destruction directed at laboratories in both the USA and Europe by animal rights activists [246] [247] [248] [249].

However much some people insist otherwise, the vast majority of experts across all disciplines overwhelmingly consider animal testing to be absolutely vital. The number of scientists who used animal testing when developing the COVID vaccine alone is incredible [250]. Every university uses animals to further their research projects. If there were other resources that were just as reliable or more economic, they would surely be welcomed by the scientific community. But currently there aren't.

The number of institutions that defend and demonstrate the necessity of animal testing is immense. The US National Association for Biomedical Research alone represents more than 360 universities [251]. Harvard and Stanford, among others, are explicitly in favour of these techniques [252] [253].

In Europe, the most prestigious universities and laboratories, such as the Pasteur Institute, the French Veterinary Academy and Sorbonne University in Paris, adopt very similar positions. So much so that, beyond the legislation, which as we shall see is very strict, the institutions that use animals are committed to being transparent and to publicly sharing what they are doing, how they are doing it, and why, as established in the transparency charter of French institutions [254] or in declarations such as the Basel Declaration, which unites the vast majority of German and Swiss medical associations and universities [255].

And this transparency is clear: for example, in Spain, any citizen can not only see the number of animals used in experiments carried out in their country, but they can also find out what species these animals belong to, how severe the procedures performed on them were, the degree of pain or distress, whether the animals are genetically modified or not, whether they are reused or not, as well as the purpose of the research – all at the click of a button on a ministry's website [256].

And so we come to the aspect that everyone must respect, and that is the legislation, which, as we said, is very strict. Anyone who wants to conduct animal testing in Europe must comply with the regulations based on Directive 2010/63/EU of the European Parliament [257], which establishes that research with animals must always be based on ethical considerations, good practices and the minimisation of animal suffering. Furthermore, all experiments must be carried out by specifically trained staff. In 1959, a group of British universities launched the idea of replacing, reducing and refining the use of animals. This concept is known as the 3Rs and can be summarised as follows:

- Replace: use cell cultures instead of live animals wherever possible.
- Reduce: minimise the number of animals required as much as possible. For example, new MRI techniques allow more information per animal to be collected, reducing the absolute number of animals required for a specific research project.
- Refine: use precise techniques to reduce animal suffering and distress. To do this, we can use anaesthetics, analgesics or less invasive techniques to obtain samples for analysis.

In the USA, the Animal Welfare Act represents the legal framework for protecting animal welfare.

The case of thalidomide is clear proof that animal testing is essential. This drug was approved to alleviate dizziness in pregnant women, but ultimately was responsible responsible for severe malformations (absence of limbs) in the babies of the women who took it. It was not approved in the USA because it was never validated as safe there as the tests needed to prove its safety had not been carried out on experimental animals [258] [259]. Tragically, this was not the case in Spain, where the product was authorised, and as a result numerous babies were born with the severe malformations described.

However much some people insist otherwise, the vast majority of experts across all disciplines overwhelmingly consider animal testing to be absolutely vital.

When a sector can stop performing animal testing, it does so. For example, the automobile industry used numerous animals from different species to develop anti-collision safety elements in vehicles. Around the end of the 1980s, once computer simulations became more accurate and dummies started to be used, the use of animals stopped completely [260].

Nevertheless, animal testing remains essential for developing new drugs and vaccines. Without these *in vivo* tests, we wouldn't today be able to discover new therapeutic solutions for a range of diseases. Proof of this is the fact that, on 11 March 2013, the European Union banned the use of animals to test compounds used in the cosmetic industry. However, as a dossier produced by the EU itself acknowledges, there are still tests that cannot be carried out *in vitro* or by computer simulations. This is one of the conclusions of the EU's own report:

"Despite considerable progress made in the development, validation and regulatory acceptance of alternative-to-animal methods, alternative test methods have not yet been accepted by the international regulatory community for the safety assessment of ingredients for some of the most complex endpoints, such as repeated dose toxicity, reproductive toxicity or carcinogenicity. Until all toxicological endpoints can be covered by alternatives, the European cosmetics industry remains limited in its ability to introduce new ingredients, apply for new uses of existing ingredients, or respond to new questions regarding the safety of existing ingredients" [261].

Animal testing remains essential for developing new drugs and vaccines. Without these *in vivo* tests, we wouldn't today be able to discover new therapeutic solutions for a range of diseases.

In any case, the cosmetics industry used a tiny fraction of all the animals used for testing within the EU, 0.05% to be precise [262]. So this regulatory change, important from a qualitative point of view, has had a very moderate impact on the quantitative aspect and shows that if we want to make further progress in fields such as toxicology, pharmacology, immunology, genetics and biochemistry, we need the help of animals. Of course, we must also minimise their discomfort and avoid their use whenever possible, as specified by legislation and common sense.

In addition to being essential for obtaining new vaccines and medicines, animal testing enables new surgical techniques to be developed. Thanks to these techniques, transplantation is now relatively frequent and safe. Thanks to the practice surgeons are able to acquire using animal models, we are able to re-implant amputated limbs, perform hip implants, and implement less invasive techniques such as laparoscopy [263].

Clearly, although legislation protects the animals used in such studies, further progress must be made in caring for them, minimising their discomfort, and paying attention to improving their quality of life. This is what some companies that need to use these animals already do. Once the tests have been completed, the animals that participated in them are adopted by families and spend the rest of their lives as pets. A French NGO, Gircor, is responsible for this scheme in coordination with a range of research institutions and companies [264] [265] [266].

PETS AND ANIMAL RIGHTS

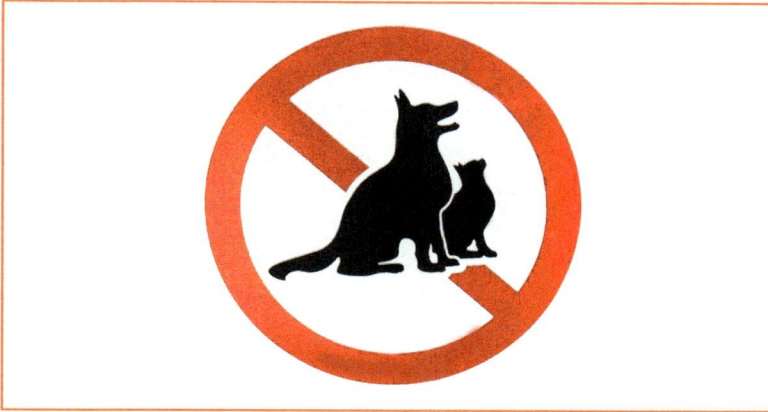

Millions of people give and receive affection to and from the millions of cats and dogs that live with them, that they care for, and from which they sometimes receive care, in the case of guide dogs for example.

In the United States, there are around 90 million dogs in households and around 60 million cats. The cost per animal per year on veterinary care alone is $253 and $98, respectively [267] [268].

Moving back to Europe, in France there are 15 million cats and more than 7 million dogs [269] [270], and in Spain the numbers are 3 million and 5 million respectively [271] [272], with an average monthly cost of €130 per dog and €90 per cat [273]. And these are the animals counted in the census, the real numbers may be higher.

I'm giving you this data to show how much interest there is in pets, how their presence is becoming more and more important – the number of adoptions increased massively during the COVID confinement – for millions of people whose lives they make happier.

However, for a growing strain of animal rights groups, ownership – this noun alone signifies a relationship of control according to these ideologues – of pets should be abolished. This is the thesis – among others – of another of the champions of the cause, namely Gary Francione, professor of law at a renowned

American university [274]. He is a fierce critic of Singer, who he accuses of being half-hearted in his defence of animals.

One of the points on which his thesis is based, you could say its cornerstone, is that animals should not be owned, because it is only moral to own things, and since animals are not things, owning them should be prohibited. He believes that this ownership is synonymous with exploitation – it would be interesting to know how the animals interpret this term or what they think of it – and, therefore, it should be ended completely by preventing domesticated animals (dogs and cats included) from reproducing.

I don't know how the millions of pets who live happily with their owners – sorry – and who have lives of the highest quality, with high quality veterinary care and who are considered as full members of the family by thousands of families would respond to this theorist. Nor does it sound very respectful to prevent every animal from following its reproductive instinct.

In addition to conjectures of varying degrees of extravagance, it's important to note that, as a species, dogs only exist in human homes or near to humans. Even stray dogs feed on waste found in rubbish dumps and are always in close proximity to people [275]. Dogs do not hunt, they eat what we give them; whether it be voluntarily at home or unintentionally in the waste we throw away. So, no matter how hard Francione tries, dogs will always be close to us and there will always be a child who will want to adopt them, and that dog will happily become part of a home.

And this is another contradiction that we frequently find in the anti-speciesist movement: a profound lack of knowledge of the animal world, of what animals' preferences are, and of their behaviour and needs. It remains a profoundly anthropocentric movement.

Nevertheless, our cats and dogs still have to face another inconvenience that puts their existence at risk. Our beloved pets eat meat. And that, of course, is a cardinal sin that some vegans cannot forgive. So, there are two alternatives: get rid of pets or get our pets to stop eating meat. Again, we come back to the animal rights movement's manifest ignorance of the animal world despite, in theory, looking out for animals' welfare.

It is mind-boggling to see how a growing number of vegan websites and articles advocate converting dogs and cats to veganism. I don't understand why a cat or dog should follow its owner's ideology. It's as absurd as me saying my dog has to support Real Madrid or Barcelona. In any case, having a pet is not obligatory. Furthermore, there are pets that are vegan by nature, rabbits and guinea pigs for example, that can be just as interesting companions as cats and dogs and who wouldn't have to be subjected to unnecessary nutritional stress. It's striking how this movement, which seeks to live in harmony with the environment, unashamedly denies pets this opportunity, because for dogs and cats, meat is fundamental.

Fundamental for various reasons. Firstly because they like it. A lot. They are devoted to it and to deny it to them is a disservice to their welfare. Secondly, although a dog could, in theory, get its nutrients from vegetables alone, in practice it would be rather more complex – and dangerous for their health. Although we have the image of dogs as animals that live with us in our homes, in reality, as we have already seen, most dogs throughout the world live close to humans, but not with them. So, millions of dogs scavenge for food in landfills on the outskirts of large cities in developing countries. In this environment, if given the choice, dogs won't eat the fruit peel or cereal grains they find in the rubbish, they'll go for any discarded meat they find. Although their digestive system can digest carbohydrates and fruits, their preference for meat is clear, as anyone who has a dog could tell you.

> It's striking how a movement that seeks to live in harmony with the environment, unashamedly denies pets this opportunity, because for dogs and cats, meat is fundamental.

For their part, although they are omnivores (even if some authors disagree with this classification and consider them carnivores [276]), dogs have a clear preference for products of animal origin. And although, theoretically, they could live on vegetables [277], dog nutrition experts are reluctant to recommend this type of diet, as it must be designed with extreme care and it is very easy for the dog to end up with nutritional deficiencies. Dogs need a lot of protein in their diet, and its not just important that it's present in their diet, it must also contain all the amino acids they need and be bioavailable. It is possible but it really is difficult and risky to try to meet all their needs with a plant-based diet. Moreover, doing this on an ongoing basis is complex and requires regular testing of the animal – as in humans – to see if its vitamin and mineral levels are correct, which does not improve its welfare. A not insignificant number of veterinarians oppose this practice [278] because, for a dog, it shouldn't be a question of surviving with a vegan diet but thriving with a diet that contains meat. The British Veterinary Association goes so far as to explicitly recommend against feeding dogs a vegan diet [279]. Of course, a diet containing dairy and meat is vital for a puppy in its growth phase.

Therefore, by feeding them a vegan diet we would be risking having dogs with compromised health [280] [281] or that are forced to behave in a way contrary to their instinct. In any case, we have to choose: cats and dogs can eat animal products, we can put their health at great risk, or we eliminate them from our society. It is as absurd to give a vegan diet to a dog as to make a horse eat meat, something which is possible in extreme circumstances but not desirable [282].

The British Veterinary Association explicitly opposes feeding dogs and cats a vegan diet.

The case of cats is even more extreme. Our cats have to eat meat. Their digestive system, unlike that of dogs, cannot digest plant starch and they must get their energy from protein, which they consume in proportionately larger quantities than dogs and humans. Furthermore, they require certain amino acids that are only found in meat. In short, subjecting a cat to a vegan diet is condemning it to death.

The studies on the issue are clear: cats need to eat a lot of protein and this must be of animal origin, because this is the only source that doesn't just contain amino acids but also contains vitamins, fats and minerals in sufficient quantities that can be absorbed by cats [283] [284] [285]. Even companies that specialise in pet food advise against vegan diets for cats [286].

However, that's not the only problem that cats present to the animal rights community. Another important aspect is the fact that every cat – if it leaves the house – is a consummate hunter [287] and this natural instinct drives them to prey on millions of birds, small mammals and reptiles. Their activity puts some ecosystems at risk. To give one example, a study in the United Kingdom found that a sample of 963 cats brought home more than fourteen thousand items of prey in five months [288].

A study in the US found that cats there hunt around 1.3 billion birds and 6 billion small mammals every year [289].

In fact, according to some animal rights activists who propose that domestic animals should have full citizenship rights – yes, you read that right – dogs and cats would have to give up eating meat, since their freedom ends where other animals' freedom to live begins. This is why these same authors go so far in their work as to flirt with the possibility of driving cats to extinction [202].

Some propose sterilising them all and others directly physically eliminating them. Others, such as the Spanish animal rights party PACMA, believe that feral cat colonies that spring up in urban areas should be defended [290], even when they put the diversity of other species at risk, as is happening to the Tenerife speckled lizard [291]. Coherence is not dogma in this movement.

To me, it seems reasonable to leave things as they are, to have our cats with us, feed them appropriately and to prevent, as far as possible, them adding a bird or rodent they've caught to their diet.

The vegan world also sees the domestication and riding of horses as abuse. Even the use of guide dogs for blind people is compared to slavery because the animal is forced to be by a person's side and to serve them without having chosen this option voluntarily [292].

Everyone can draw their own conclusions, but in a fully vegan world with full animal rights there would be no cats, dogs would be profoundly unhappy, and horses would have to go back to galloping free on the prairies. Incidentally, we can see the consequences of such a situation in the USA, where feral horses or *mustangs* have become a plague and a real environmental problem [293] [294].

II

ENVIRONMENTAL REASONS: VEGANISM AND THE ENVIRONMENT

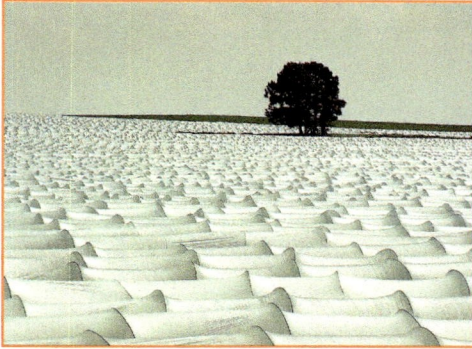

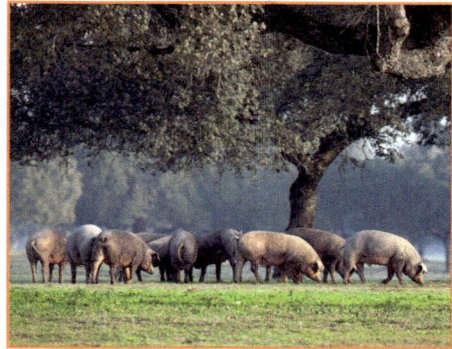

Sometimes, the production of vegetables is not environmentally friendly. Seas of plastic, necessary for certain crops, contrast with some livestock farming practices linked to the land.

The lengths that some supporters of the vegan cause will go to, in order to communicate their belief that animal production inflicts all kinds of ills on the health of the planet, are striking. Most notable, they argue, is its negative effect on the environment in general and climate change – or greenhouse gases (GHGs) – in particular.

In addressing issues such as animal consciousness or the morality of animal husbandry, we addressed ideas that, although well founded and argued, leave room for opinion. Science today doesn't have all the answers and, as a result, particularly on questions of morality, there will be opinions and streams of thought to accommodate different positions on these issues.

However, the environmental question finds strong support in the science community and therefore, the debate – should it be necessary – should at least be considered and based on the high quantity of verified data that we have available.

137

LIVESTOCK AND GREENHOUSE GASES (GHGS)

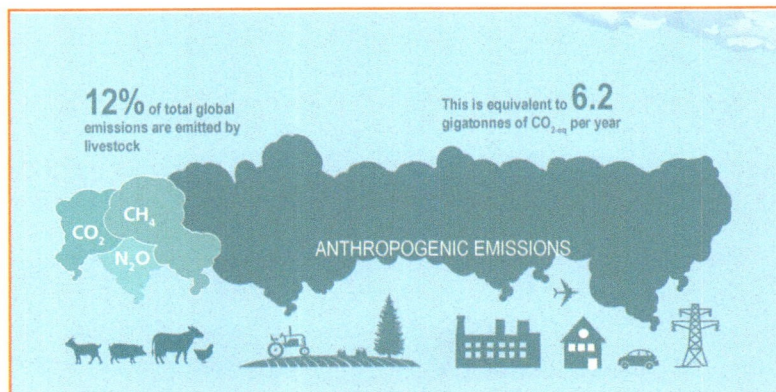

12% of total global emissions are emitted by livestock

This is equivalent to 6.2 gigatonnes of CO_{2-eq} per year

CO_2 CH_4 N_2O

ANTHROPOGENIC EMISSIONS

Emissions of animal origin – both direct and indirect – represent 12% of total global emissions.

Source: © FAO Global Livestock Environmental Assessment Model. Livestock solutions for climate change. Global Livestock Environmental Assessment Model (GLEAM) | Food and Agriculture Organization of the United Nations (fao.org)

Animal rights organisations' publications often refer to the impact that livestock farming has on global warming. In this field, we have the huge advantage of having objective measurements of the impact of different industries and a global reference accepted by the scientific community – the IPCC, the Intergovernmental Panel on Climate Change. This organisation was created in 1988 by two UN agencies, namely the World Meteorological Organization and the United Nations Environment Programme. The IPCC prepares reports that contribute to the work of the United Nations Framework Convention on Climate Change (UN-FCCC), the main international agreement on climate change. The objective of the UNFCCC is the "stabilization of greenhouse gas concentrations in the atmosphere at a level that would prevent dangerous anthropogenic [i.e., human-caused] interference with the climate system". For example, the Fifth Assessment Report of the IPCC was a scientific work critical of the UNFCCC's 2015 Paris Agreement.

The IPCC is the global reference on the contribution of different industries and natural phenomena to the production of GHGs. Its reports are based on reference material from experts in a range of subjects and it also collects data from other organisations, such as the FAO.

The data published by the IPCC and, in this case, collected by the FAO indicates that, of total human-induced greenhouse gas emissions, i.e. emissions caused by various human activities, animal production accounts for 14.5% (this data includes direct emissions (5%) and indirect emissions) [295].

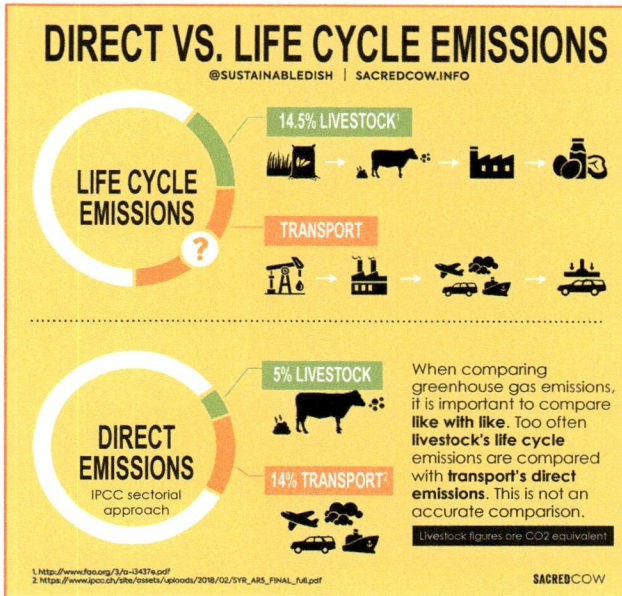

Direct emissions from livestock (gases emitted by animals) account for 5% of total global emissions, while direct emissions from transport (exhaust gases) account for 14%. If we combine direct and indirect (from tractors, feed factories, etc.) emissions, livestock contributes a total of 14.5% (similar to transport direct emissions alone), while the indirect emissions from transport have not been measured. It's therefore very important that we compare equivalent emissions so we can see which sector emits the most.

It's clear that emissions are a factor that the sector should try to reduce, but it's also clear that the use of fossil fuels is, by far, the main source of GHGs.

And not all livestock species emit the same amount of gases nor do all production systems emit GHGs in the same way. In fact the IPCC reports that pigs [295] and poultry only contribute a total of 1.3% and 1.5% of all global emissions respectively and fish farming accounts for a mere 0.5%.

Let's look at some examples that will help us understand this point:

Emissions generated by livestock within the European Union (EU) account for 5.8% of the total [296]. On the other hand, emissions from animal production in the United States account for around 4% [297].

On the other hand, if we look at regions like Latin America, with total livestock production numbers similar to Europe, we see that they generate double the GHGs of the EU. If we look at another region, such as South Asia, the livestock production output (total protein produced) is less than half of the protein produced in Europe, however the emissions are slightly higher than they are in Europe [298].

Western Europe has the highest milk production in the world and the lowest emissions from its production.

This is because the efficiency of production is key to reducing emissions. For example, to produce the same quantity of milk as one USA cow, you would need 5 cows in Mexico and 20 in India. In North America, the dairy cattle population has dropped from 12 million in 1970 to 9 million today, yet milk production has tripled. Thanks to genetic, nutritional and health improvements, the animals produce more and, therefore, the percentage of emissions per kilo or litre of end product has decreased [299].

Western Europe has the highest milk production in the world and the lowest emissions per kg.

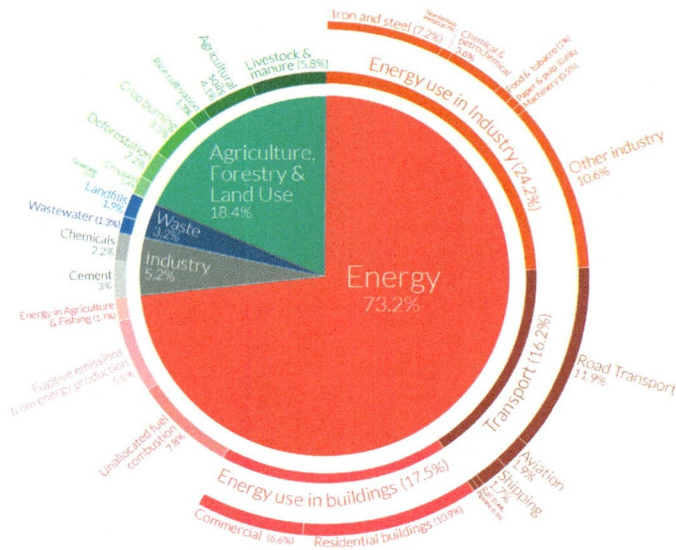

Where do global greenhouse gas emissions come from?
Source: https://ourworldindata.org/ghg-emissions-by-sector

We can, therefore, conclude that livestock farming, like all activity, causes GHGs but it is far from being one of the main sources of them.

Also, we should consider the case of India – the second highest emitter of methane globally [300]. It has more than 300 million cows, the majority unproductive but still making a significant contribution to total livestock emissions. These animals are kept in a state of low productivity for social and religious reasons, which must be respected. However, perhaps international organisations should account for their GHG emissions differently, because attributing them to livestock farming does not reflect their *raison d'être*.

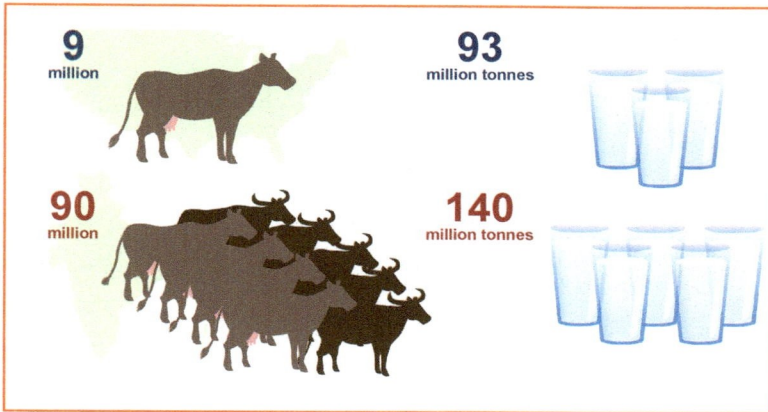

Each dairy cow in the USA produces more than 10 tonnes of milk per year. In India, the average production is 1.5 tonnes per cow per year. Increasing their productivity would reduce the emissions per kilogram of milk.

Source: The innovation revolution in agriculture. A roadmap to value creation
http://creativecommons.org/licenses/by/4.0/

We cannot get a full picture of emissions from cattle without bearing some additional data in mind.

- Firstly, we count emissions as if livestock herds had come from nothing. However ruminant animals, whether domesticated or wild, have always populated every continent and, according to calculations published by the University of Oxford [301], GHG emissions from animal sources have been as high or higher in previous eras than they are today.
- A practical and relatively well documented example of this are the emissions that bison herds produced in North America before the arrival of Europeans. When the first Europeans reached the land that is now the USA, the bison population numbered 50–80 million animals [302]. The massacre of these animals took them to the brink of extinction and today, although they are no

longer at risk, their numbers are still low. Emissions by ruminants bred for meat or milk are not that different to the emissions from the original ruminants that were living there when the settlers arrived. If the reverse phenomena occurred, i.e. if we eliminated or greatly reduced the number of grazing animals, their space would be taken up by wild ungulates [303] and total emissions would probably remain unchanged.

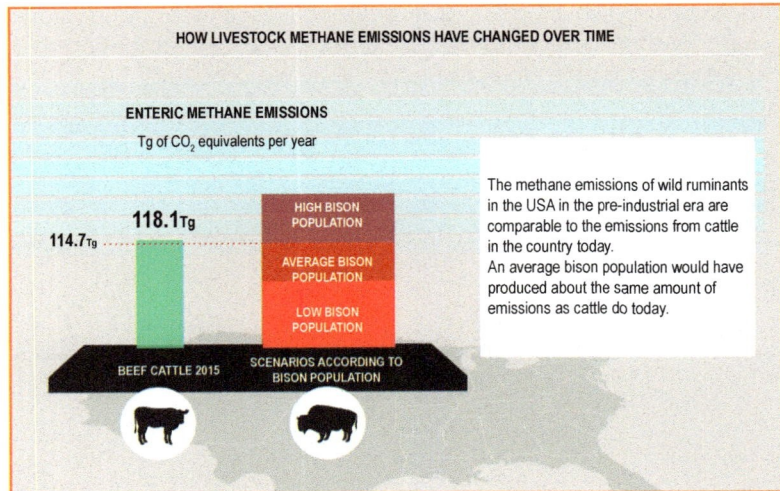

Source: Reuter, R., M. Beck, and L. Thompson. 2020. "Tough Questions About Beef Sustainability: What are Enteric Methane Emissions?" Beef Research Enteric Methane Emissions (beefresearch.org).

We therefore must differentiate between emissions of animal origin that, although they have increased as the number of animals has increased in direct proportion to the global population, have always been emitted, and fossil fuel emissions that were non-existent until we started exploiting these fuels at the start of the Industrial Revolution.

Based on this data, several authors conclude that adopting a diet completely free of products of animal origin would reduce total GHG emissions by around 2–3% in both the USA [304] and Europe [305] once the appropriate corrections have been made. The protein and energy these products provide would have to be replaced by plant products, and the production of these products also generates GHG emissions which need to be considered in the calculations.

Furthermore, some authors claim that a vegan diet would be cheaper for families. However, this potential saving would be invested in products whose manufacture may result in more emissions than the production of meat, milk and eggs. Therefore, the net result could be worse than if we consumed products of animal origin [306].

On similar lines, a study performed in 60,000 homes in Japan [307] did not find that carbon footprints were higher in homes where meat consumption was higher. Instead, the highest carbon footprints were driven by clothing consumption, eating out and alcohol consumption.

We started our description of GHG emissions of animal origin and their quantification by the FAO, which puts them at 12% of total direct and indirect emissions [308].

However, there is one factor we must consider that could cause the IPCC to modify this figure in the future, as a study from the University of Oxford explains [309]. To measure the impact of a gas on atmospheric warming, it is compared to the reference gas, which is CO_2. Thus methane (CH_4), which is the gas that animals (especially ruminants) emit through their belching, is compared with carbon dioxide. Methane traps heat with an effectiveness 28 times greater than CO_2. Therefore, the impact of CH_4 is considered to be 28 times greater than that of CO_2. However, as the experts from the renowned British university make clear, this calculation doesn't factor in the important fact that CH_4 has an atmospheric lifetime of around 10 years, while CO_2 remains in the atmosphere for centuries.

In fact, in its latest report the IPCC [310] recognises that equating 100-year methane emissions with CO_2 emissions may have resulted in errors when quantifying the weight of methane emissions in total emissions.

Some authors claim that a vegan diet would be cheaper for families. However, this potential saving would be invested in products whose manufacture could result in more emissions than the production of meat, milk and eggs. Therefore, the net result could be worse than if we consumed products of animal origin.

And what does methane turn into after 10 years? Into CO_2, but we'll see later that this CO_2 of animal origin has a smaller impact on global warming because it forms part of the carbon cycle, which is a natural cycle that has been broken by the arrival of fossil fuels. To illustrate this, we need to understand that the methane emitted by cows comes from the grass they eat; grass that has absorbed CO_2 in order to grow. When the animal digests this grass, part of its cellulose is converted into methane, which in 10 years is converted back into CO_2. Other plants will use this gas to grow and remove it from the atmosphere, and the cycle continues. So, CO_2 of animal origin forms part of the carbon cycle and will be captured by grasses and plants, which in turn will be eaten by other ruminants, thus closing the cycle. The CO_2 we emit when we breathe is measured in the same way [311].

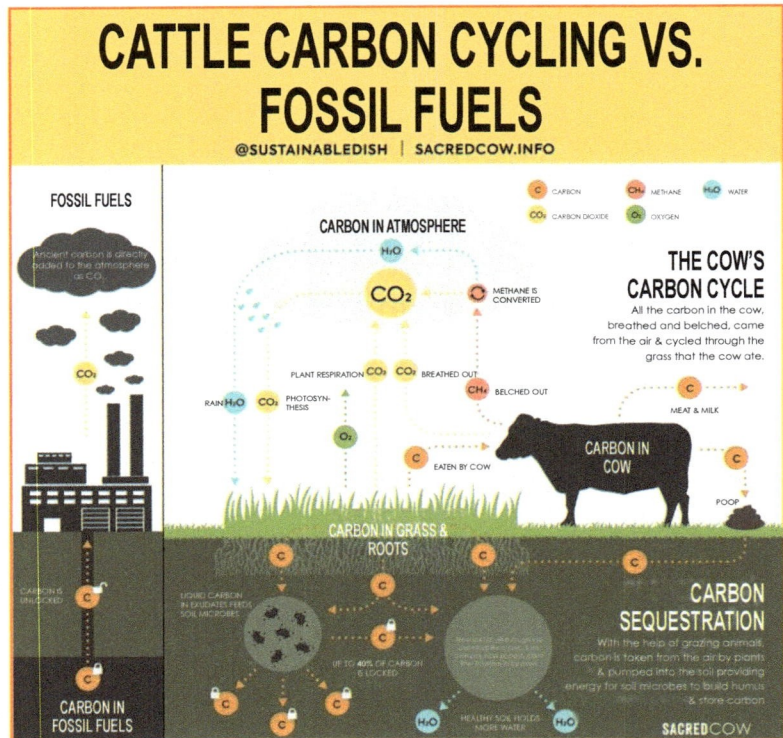

In contrast, fossil fuels have been buried for millions of years, and once the CO_2 that comes with their use is released, it is not part of any cycle. The planet does not have sufficient resources to absorb this gas the way it does the emissions of animal origin [312].

Another factor that should be studied further, but which is not considered when assessing the negative impact that cattle could have, is these animals' capacity to increase the amount of carbon dioxide that a pasture captures, in other words removes from the atmosphere. The data regarding this is very variable, given that there are a lot of factors that determine how much carbon dioxide soil or pasture can capture. However, it's logical to think that wherever livestock graze, the growth of the grass is stimulated and therefore it must capture more CO_2 from the atmosphere. Furthermore, the animals' faeces help trap the carbon in the soil [313] [314].

Therefore, we can conclude that livestock activity, like every other activity, has an impact on the environment but that it is a relatively minor GHG emitter and its impact is probably overestimated. Furthermore, the alternative of giving up animal products is not a very attractive proposition because, as we have seen, it could result in a bigger impact on the environment. Homes that do not eat animal products do not emit less greenhouse gases and, lastly, as we will discuss later, vegetable waste is much higher than waste from products of animal origin.

Fossil fuels have been buried for millions of years, and once the CO_2 that comes with their emission is released, it is not part of any cycle. The planet does not have sufficient resources to absorb this gas, but it does for the emissions of animal origin.

Ultimately, even the environmental NGO Greenpeace [315] [316] has acknowledged that pollution decreased very significantly during the COVID pandemic lockdown. The data suggests that this was the case all over the world [317]. It must be remembered that the number of farm animals animals did not reduce during this period, however transportation went down sharply, which goes to show that fossil fuels and not animals are the biggest contributor to GHG emissions.

The aspects we have looked at in this chapter prove that the consumption of products of animal origin has a moderate impact and that this impact could be reduced even further by making the animals more productive. However, I intend to go a step further and present data indicating that giving up these products would be suicidal from a social, ecological, environmental and health perspective and, therefore, that eliminating animals completely from our diet would not merely be morally questionable, it would be clearly morally reprehensible.

It's important to remember that some plant-based products also have a very high carbon footprint [318] [319], much higher than that of some products of animal origin. Therefore, plant-based diets are not necessarily better in terms of GHG emissions than diets containing meat, especially if the plant-based food has been frozen or transported by aeroplane.

EMISSIONS AND NUTRITIONAL DENSITY [320]

Another fallacy that is often used as an argument by people who would prefer to eliminate livestock farming rather than try to improve it, relates to the quantity of greenhouse gas emissions per kilogram of food product. In this comparison, products of animal origin generate significantly more emissions than products of plant origin. However, this approach ignores the fact that not all kilos are the same. When we apply the same logic but measure calories instead of kilograms of food product, the result is very different.

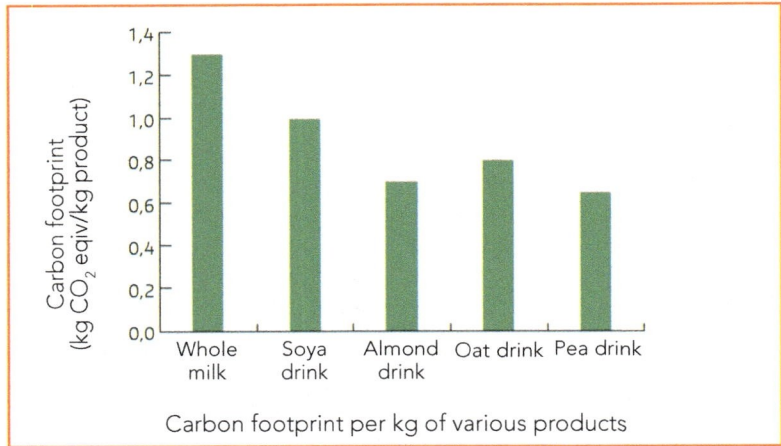

Carbon footprint per kg of various products

Clearly a kilo of carrots does not have as many calories as a kilo of meat. The kilo of meat provides more calories, as well as numerous other nutrients such as vitamins, minerals and amino acids. Let's take, for example, cow's milk and the so-called plant-based alternatives. We can see that, measured by the kilogram, the emissions from milk are higher. However, when we measure these same emissions based on the quality of nutrients in each, we see that cow's milk emits the least. Why? Because to obtain the same quantity and quality of nutrients with the alternatives, we would need to consume a much greater quantity, which would also generate much higher emissions.

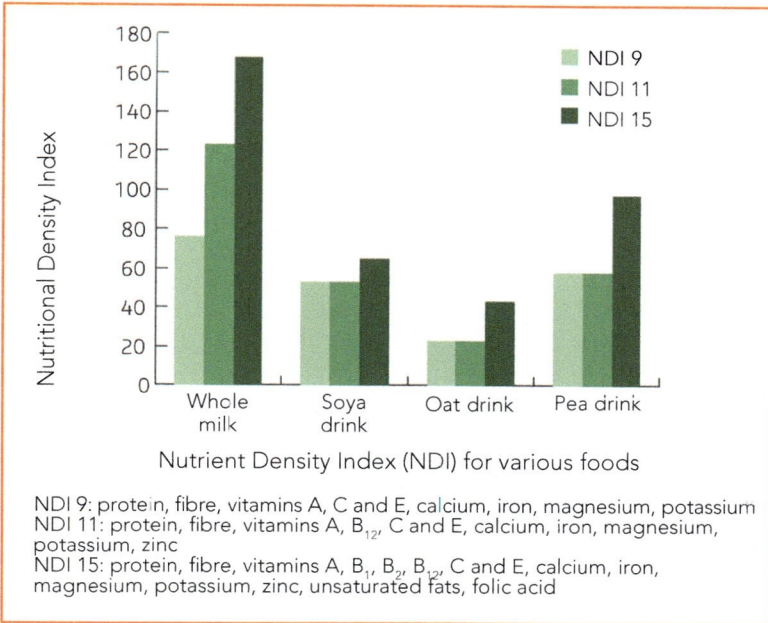

Nutrient Density Index (NDI) for various foods

NDI 9: protein, fibre, vitamins A, C and E, calcium, iron, magnesium, potassium
NDI 11: protein, fibre, vitamins A, B_{12}, C and E, calcium, iron, magnesium, potassium, zinc
NDI 15: protein, fibre, vitamins A, B_1, B_2, B_{12}, C and E, calcium, iron, magnesium, potassium, zinc, unsaturated fats, folic acid

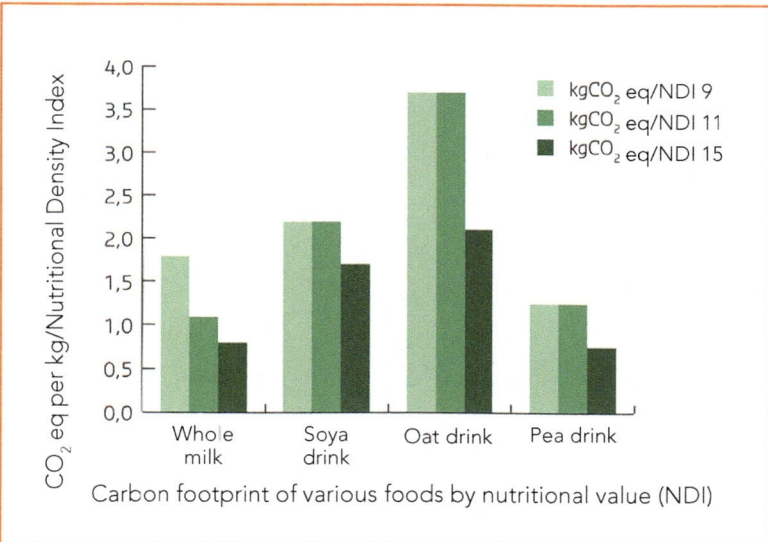

Carbon footprint of various foods by nutritional value (NDI)

Source: © Voeding Magazine 2, 2021/Dutch Dairy Association

So, we can see that happily giving up products of animal origin in our diets is not something we can – or should – do without significant consequences.

FOOD WASTE

According to the global data collected by Statista [321], 85% of food waste, i.e. food that ends up in the bin, is of plant origin. The 2018 data from the Spanish Ministry of Agriculture shows a similar trend, with fruit and vegetable products at the top of the food waste table [322] [323].

Furthermore, an interesting study [324] performed by the US Department of Agriculture together with the University of Vermont found that 51% of all fruit, vegetables and cereals bought in the USA end up in the bin, either because of selection by wholesalers or as a consequence of household waste. For meat, in contrast, only 14% ends up as waste. Each person throws out 422 g of food per day, of which 227 g is plant waste. Therefore, it is more than a bit of a leap to conclude that a vegan diet would lead to a reduction in greenhouse gas emissions given the waste it generates.

We also must remember that fruit and vegetables produced in greenhouses may emit more gases than products of animal origin [325]. This is also the case if the plant-based food is transported by aeroplane [326] [327].

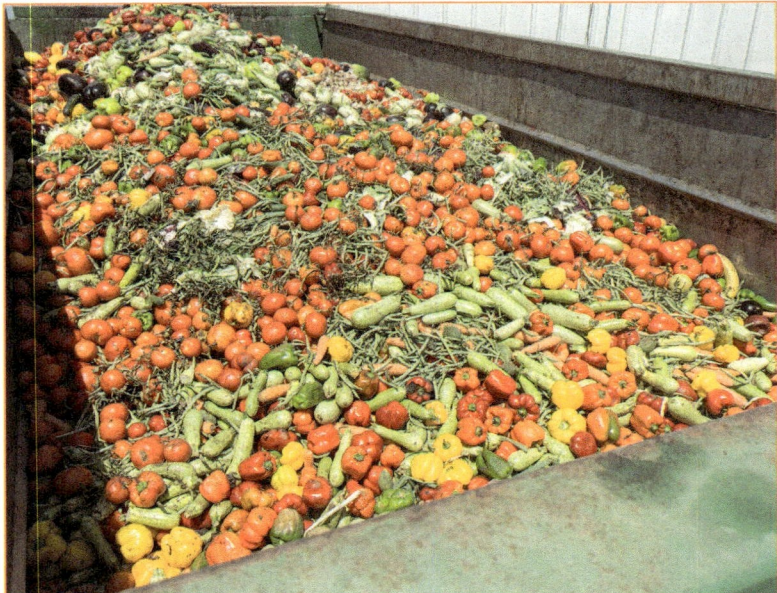

ANIMAL PRODUCTION AND THE USE OF AGRICULTURAL LAND

You often see activist organisations that are in favour of plant-based diets argue that breeding animals means taking a huge amount of nutrients out of our diet that we could consume directly, avoiding the middleman (livestock). They say we would have more fruit and vegetables available to us and we could avoid the consumption of animals with all the evils that, according to them, this entails.

Again, let's look at the data to see the reality.

The earth's total land surface area [328] is 13.2 billion hectares, of which almost 5 billion is used for agriculture and livestock farming (today we cultivate 1.6 billion hectares) and another 3.5 billion are grassland or scrubland that would be difficult to utilise if livestock were not grazing on it [329]. In other words, the amount of land we use, either for cultivation or pasture-raised livestock is approximately one hundred times the surface of Spain.

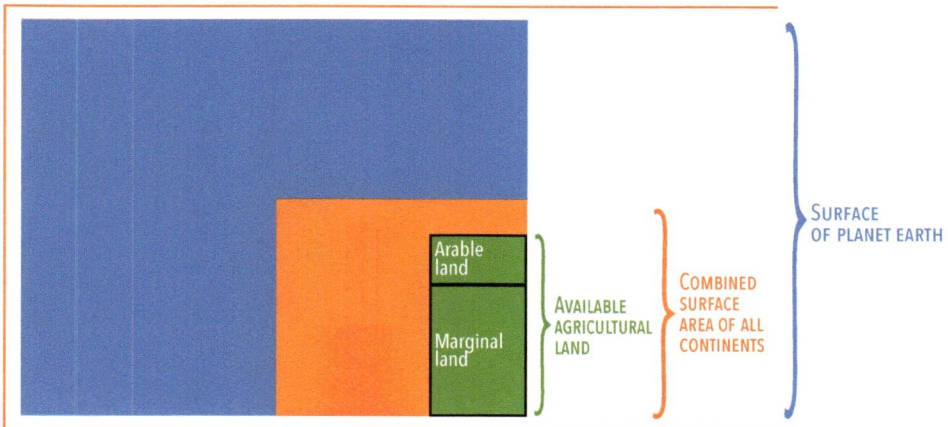

However, it's important to clarify that, although a significant part of the planet's available land is used for livestock, we must remember that it's the only way we have to sustainably use this land and to contribute to the food security of millions of people around the world. Two thirds of the world's agricultural land is marginal land that cannot be cultivated, because it is of poor quality, has low rainfall, is mountainous or is semi-desert.

The only way of getting anything out of such land is with animals – above all ruminants – that are capable are transforming a few weeds into protein (milk and meat) of high nutritional quality [330].

I wonder why there is such emphasis on the area devoted to animal feed when the area devoted to perfectly dispensable crops is completely ignored? Such dispensable crops include the cereals used in the distillation of spirits or for biodiesel (up to 40% of US corn production [331]), the area devoted to tobacco, cannabis, teas, coffee, yerba mate, vines and ornamental plants, to name but a few. Following the same logic, eliminating these crops would allow us to return millions of square kilometres to nature so it can be inhabited by wild flora and fauna. Of course, I wouldn't defend this alternative, but it surprises me that the people who disdain and attack livestock farming don't show the same level of aggressiveness and opposition to these crops which, however pleasant they may be, don't provide anything vital to our survival. They certainly provide much less than products of animal origin.

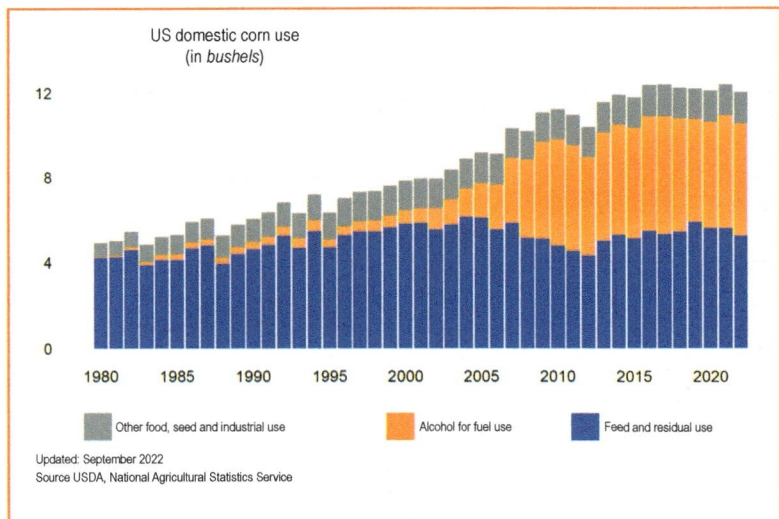

US domestic corn use
(in *bushels*)

Other food, seed and industrial use   Alcohol for fuel use   Feed and residual use

Updated: September 2022
Source USDA, National Agricultural Statistics Service

We have to be very clear here because, although the argument has inherent logic, as the French poet and essayist Jean Cocteau said "A half empty bottle of wine is also half full, but half a lie will never be half true".

THE *RAISON D'ETRE* OF LIVESTOCK

To start off, it's important to understand why humans started farming livestock. This qualitative leap that allowed man to tame plants and animals, and which gave rise to the Neolithic period, allowed settlement in towns and villages, gave humans enough time to devote to tasks other than getting their daily sustenance and, in short, allowed the development of trades, writing, art and science.

Why did the first people who decided to feed and care for animals want to do this? We'll see that the original reason isn't that different from our current reasons, albeit with some caveats. There is a very important basic idea behind livestock farming: transforming the inedible into edible food. Animals have always recycled what we cannot eat and, as we shall see, still do: from a meadow where cows graze, a flock of sheep that eats the stubble left after the harvest, a pig that will eat wormy tubers, fruit skins or eggshells, to chickens that will gladly eat worms from the ground or the carcass of an animal.

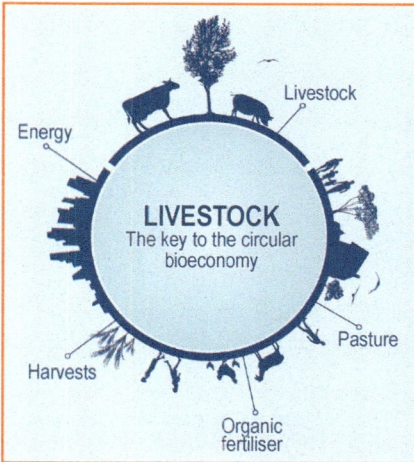

Livestock recycles resources that otherwise would be lost because only animals can use them. In return, we get top quality nutrients and manure that will make the fields more fertile or that we can use to make biogas. A perfect example of a circular economy.

© 2016 Inge Milou Krijger for ATF

Today, their role hasn't changed that much. According to data from the FAO [332], globally domesticated animals consume around 6 billion metric tonnes of feed every year. This data is very important as it shows that 86% of everything that livestock consumes globally is composed of grasses and other plant debris that humans cannot digest directly. Grasses and leaves consumed by animals – especially ruminants – account for 46% of this total.

The rest is a mix of multiple by-products from a range of industries whose waste is used by livestock. This means that without livestock's contribution, they would have to be discarded and would create a major environmental problem, as they would either rot – with the resulting pollution – or they would have to be destroyed – which would also mean transporting and burning them. Either of these solutions would undoubtedly have a high environmental cost. For example, we would have to deal with what remains after the sugar has been extracted from sugar beet or sugar cane, peel from fruit used to make juices, industrial brewery waste, cottonseed, corn stalks, stubble left over after cereals have been harvested, sunflower and other oilseed cakes after the oil has been extracted, and we could name hundreds more. We also have to take into account that this study by the FAO does not include other products that livestock recycles, such as serums and other waste from the dairy and cheese industry, plasma, blood serums and other waste from slaughterhouses, such as feathers and rumen content, meat meal and poultry litter.

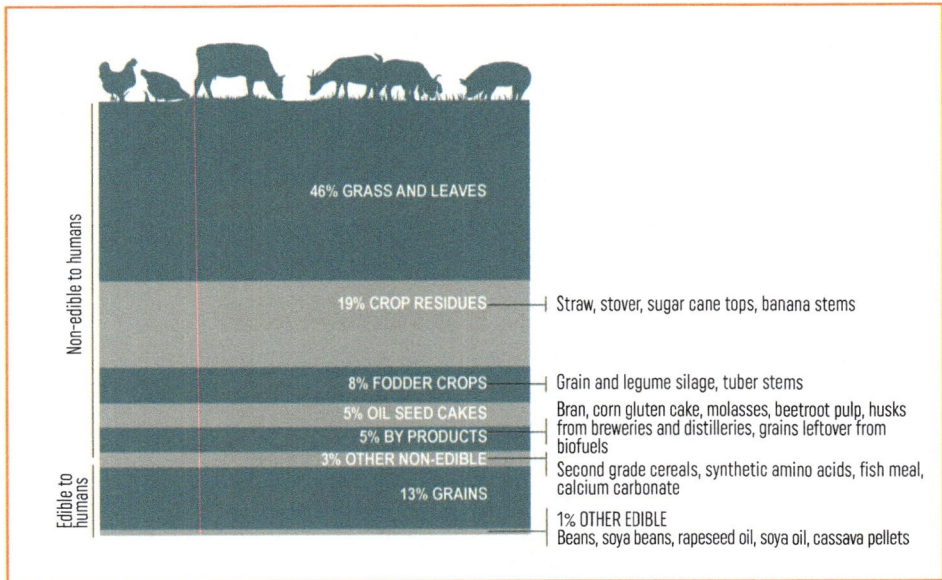

Pasture and sub-products that we cannot digest account for 86% of the food livestock consumes.

Source: © FAO 2022 More Fuel for the Food/Feed Debate More fuel for the food/feed debate (fao.org)

In fact, for every 0.6 kg of human-usable protein we give them, cattle give us back 1 kg of digestible protein. How is this possible? Because they are capable of eating and digesting vegetable by-products that we cannot, but which are very nutritious for them [332].

So we see that, from remains of no value and with no other use, animals manage to provide us with their own products rich in proteins and other nutrients or with their strength (not an insignificant aspect in some underdeveloped countries) and other animal by-products that are used in a range of industries and which, on most occasions, go unnoticed. Livestock recycles.

For example [333] the majority of glues and adhesives, as well as a lot of paints and varnishes, are produced from bones. They are also used to produce explosives, fertilisers, paper, photographic film, x-ray film, cements and matches. Bones are also used in the textile industry and to manufacture porcelain, among many other things. From the skin we obtain sweets and confectionery, cosmetic collagen, clothing, plastic sheets for practising tattoos, chewing gum, beauty masks, gelatins, ice cream, beer, fruit juices and medicine capsules. From the intestines we get heparin, pancreatic insulin and heart valves for heart surgery and, from the blood, cigarette filters.

From the fat, we get soap, lubricants, biodiesel, detergent, fabric softener, paint, cosmetics, antifreeze, fertilisers and paint brushes.

Without animals, all these products – and many more – would have to be produced from other resources. Those processes would emit a lot of a gases and generate large amounts of waste.

Livestock consume plant remains and, in addition to foods of extraordinary biological value that taste great, provide us with a range of by-products that save us from a lot of productive processes.

Would it be moral to dispense with these plant and animal remains? Their use enables recycling and makes meat, milk and eggs more affordable and available to millions of people. In developed countries it may seem banal to a lot of people, but in many arid regions, having a herd of goats grazing on the four weeds growing on a rocky outcrop is a guarantee of life. It means having access to key protein for your family and your children's growth. The first world may be able to easily move on from these products (although we have seen how many vegans give up on the diet, so this assertion might be a bit bold) but for millions of people throughout the world, their availability allows them to make the most of their resources and have a reliable source of good food, which is hugely appreciated by the majority of humanity.

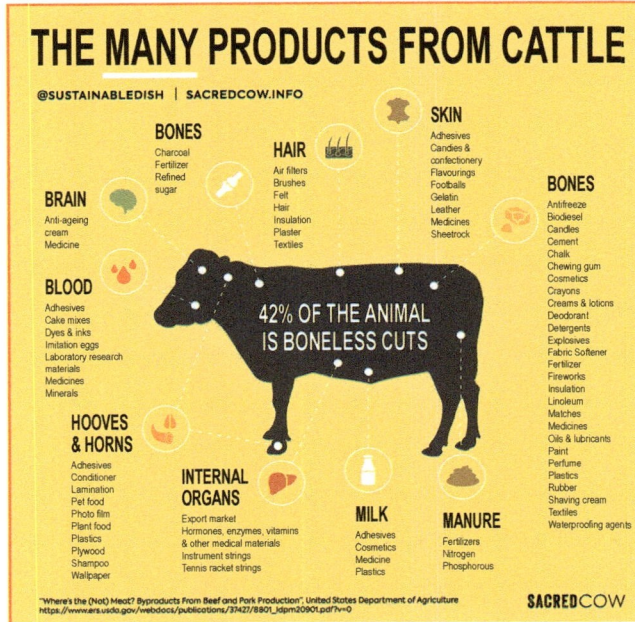

Infographic with the non-food uses of the various organs of cattle. Only 42% of the animal is boneless meat, but the whole animal is used by several different industries.

LIVESTOCK AND DEFORESTATION

Another source of frequent attacks on the livestock sector is based on the trite argument that the cultivation of soya beans uses up vast areas of the planet (particularly in the Amazon) and this is a product we could eat directly, eliminating the intermediary, which in this case is livestock.

It should be noted that while the Amazon is undergoing deforestation, the planet as a whole is being reforested, as shown by NASA satellite images [334].

Since 1990, forested areas have increased by 10% in Europe as a whole, and 30% in Spain [335].

But back to soya beans; let's look at how this pulse is used worldwide: approximately 15% is consumed directly by humans in the form of tofu, soy sauce, edamame, etc.

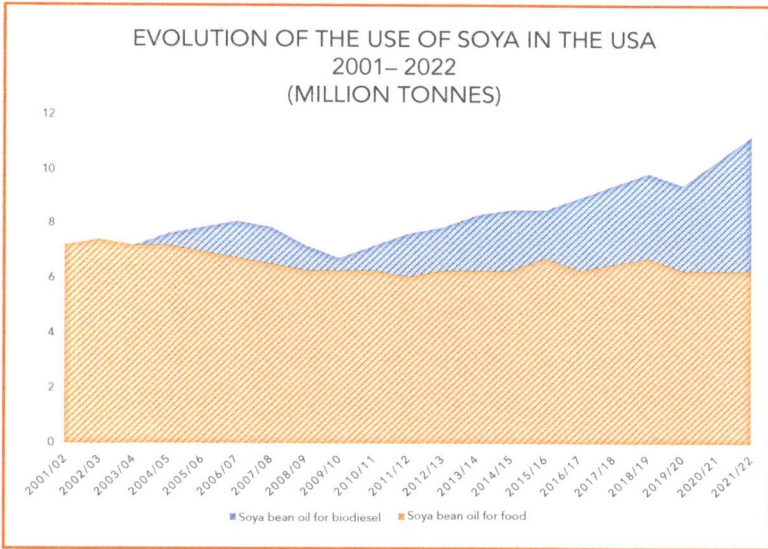

EVOLUTION OF THE USE OF SOYA IN THE USA
2001– 2022
(MILLION TONNES)

■ Soya bean oil for biodiesel   ■ Soya bean oil for food

The remaining 85% is crushed. It is crushed to obtain soyabean oil, which is the second most used cooking oil worldwide (all fast-food chains use it), and is also used in numerous industries, such as the food industry, as well as to produce paints, varnishes and biodiesel. Once the oil has been extracted, we are left with the soya cake. This cake is rich in protein and is what is fed to animals, particularly chickens and pigs. This cake would not be used if it wasn't fed to livestock. If livestock don't eat it, the soya bean waste would have to be disposed of – it might be edible but there's currently no culinary demand for the product.

The price per kilo of oil is higher than the price of the cake, although the volume of production of the latter is higher. We can therefore conclude that blaming livestock alone for the negative consequences of consuming soybeans is not a fair reflection of reality, given that livestock contributes to solving a problem. Poultry and pigs depend on soybeans as a source of protein, but numerous other industries also use it, including some that use large quantities to make biodiesel. It is also important to note that, once the oil has been used for frying in every fast-food chain in the world, some of this oil, now unusable, is used as a component of feed for... livestock! [336] [337]

We can conclude this section by stating that, as we can see from information and data from international organisations such as the FAO, banning the farming and use of animals would have devastating consequence, since billions of tonnes of plant resources left over from our food would not be recycled. There would be little gain in crop acreage, as much of what livestock eats is pasture on marginal land where agriculture does not bear fruit. We would no longer have medicines we get from animals, which are vital for many people, and we would also lose the capacity to obtain modern and effective treatments as we would not be able to test these products on animals. And all this without an appreciable benefit to the environment since, as we have seen, the impact of livestock on the generation of GHGs is minor and livestock provides a lot of elements (apart from the obvious food) that would otherwise have to be produced chemically.

III

VEGANISM AND HEALTH

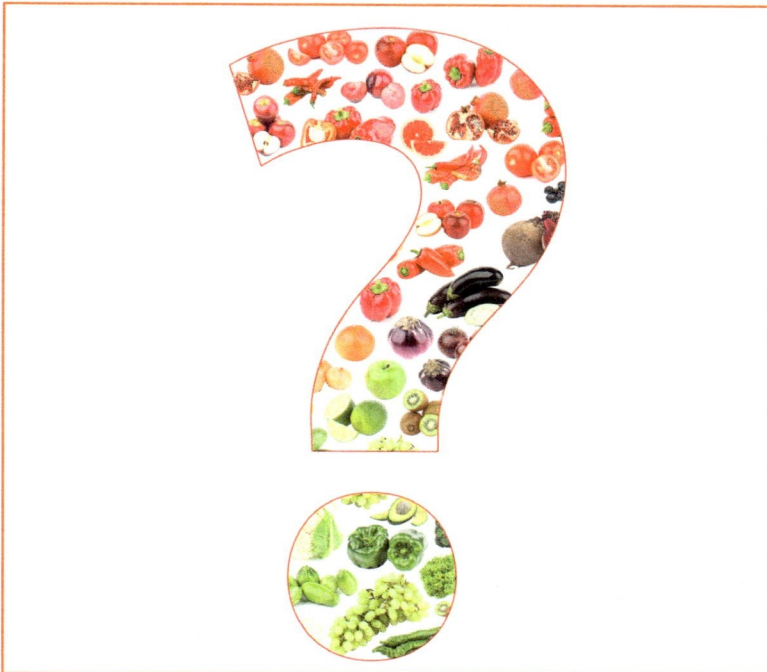

ANIMALS, HEALTH AND FOOD SECURITY

Clearly it is possible to follow a vegan diet with a total absence of food derived from animals. We have already seen how a very low percentage of people decide to take up this diet and we have also seen how the majority give it up fairly quickly. On the other hand, the data shows that a lot of self-described vegans break the rules of the diet on a regular basis. So, it's clear that it's not easy to follow through with this dietary choice.

Choosing to be vegan is a relatively recent option. Although there have been vegetarians since ancient times, the possibility of supplementing the diet with artificial additives containing the vitamins and minerals absent – or not absorbable –– from a plant-based diet has made it possible to totally eliminate animals from diets.

These supplements are produced by genetically modified bacteria or yeast and must be taken regularly to avoid deficiencies of nutrients that are key to a healthy life.

Nevertheless, there are more than a few medical and dietary organisations that, although they do not prohibit the vegan diet directly, are reticent to fully accept it – or even expressly advise against it – particularly for pregnant women, children and adolescents. So, for example:

- Belgian Superior Health Council. It warns of the risk of various nutritional deficiencies (protein, DHA, vitamins D and B_{12}, iron, zinc, iodine and calcium). It advises against these diets in pregnant and breastfeeding women and in their children under 3 years of age [338].
- European Society for Paediatric Gastroenterology, Hepatology, and Nutrition. Quote: "Vegan diets have generally been discouraged… [because]… the risks of failing to follow advice [regarding supplementation] are severe, including irreversible cognitive damage from vitamin B_{12} deficiency, and death [339]".
- German Society of Nutrition. Quote: "We do not recommend a vegan diet during pregnancy or while lactating, or during childhood or adolescence [340]".
- German Society of Paediatric and Adolescent Medicine. Quote: "A vegan diet is disadvised during all periods with intense growth and development [341]."
- Belgian Royal Academy of Medicine. Quote: "The vegan diet is not suitable for pregnant women, infants, children and adolescents and therefore cannot be recommended [342]"
- Swiss Federal Commission for Nutrition Quote: "A vegan diet cannot be recommended at a general population level, particularly critical are children, pregnant women and older adults [343]"
- Spanish Association of Paediatrics Quote: "Although following a vegetarian diet at any stage of infancy is not necessarily unsafe, it is preferable to advise that an omnivorous or at least an ovo-vegetarian or lacto-vegetarian diet should be followed during the breastfeeding period and in young children [344]".
- North American Society for Pediatric Gastroenterology, Hepatology, and Nutrition. Quote: "So-called plant-based

milks are inappropriate substitutes for children given that milk is an important part of their diet [345]".

- Danish health authorities. Quote: "The position of the society is to advise against a vegan diet during pregnancy and lactation". The Danish National Health Authorities advised parents to avoid a vegan diet when feeding young children [346].
- French Association for Paediatric Gastroenterology, Hepatology, and Nutrition. Quote: "This type of diet, which does not provide all the micronutrient requirements, exposes children to nutritional deficiencies. These can have serious consequences, especially when this diet is introduced at an early age, a period of significant growth and neurological development. Even if deficiencies have less impact on older children and adolescents, they are not uncommon and consequently should also be prevented [347]".
- Food Safety Authority of Ireland. Underlines the importance of a diet that contains animal products and advises against the use of plant-based milks in children [348].
- The Italian Society for Preventative and Social Paediatrics, the Italian Federation of Paediatricians and the Italian Society of Perinatal Medicine. Quote: "Vegan and vegetarian diets are insufficient for correct neuropsychomotor development in children as the lack of vitamin B_{12}, iron and docosahexaenoic acid may cause irreversible harm. In addition, these diets do not provide the necessary quantities of calcium and vitamin D [349].

And while it is true that many other dietary bodies do not advise against this type of diet, in some cases there is a clear conflict of interest, either because their most prominent members are vegetarians, or because they belong to religious groups that adhere to this type of diet [350].

In addition to specific recommendations, all nutritional and medical associations insist that a vegan or vegetarian diet must be well-planned and boosted with various supplements to avoid suffering deficiencies. In other words, it's a risky diet, especially for the most vulnerable: children, pregnant and breastfeeding women, etc.

I would therefore like to draw attention to the fact that adopting the diet entails risks and is infeasible in many regions of the planet. Therefore, its implementation would be a huge challenge for millions of people, a challenge with profoundly negative consequences.

The scientific evidence is clear with regard to the essential nutrients whose absence from a diet, or presence in insufficient quantities, poses a risk when following a strict vegetarian diet. It is not my intention to compile an exhaustive list, but simply to point out that the safety of these diets is more than questionable.

A HEALTHY, GLOBAL VEGAN DIET?

We have already seen how a vegan diet requires planning and precautions that the vast majority of healthy omnivores don't have to worry about [351]. There are more than a few supplements vegans have to keep at hand, since food produced from animals provides numerous amino acids, vitamins and minerals that are more difficult to get through food solely of plant origin. We can overcome all these inconveniences in the West. All the supplements, particularly vitamin B_{12}, are easy to find online or in shops as and when they are needed. Without forgetting the cost and inconvenience of taking these supplements and the frequent lab tests required to confirm that blood vitamin and mineral levels are satisfactory, we can nevertheless conclude that they are not insurmountable hurdles to following a vegan diet.

But, what about rural populations in less developed countries where these supplements are not available or are too expensive for the general population? How would populations who can only get certain nutrients from animal products deal with this new faith?

You don't have to have a great imagination to understand the consequences. India is a country where, for religious reasons, a very broad social stratum, consumes very little meat. As a result, particularly in women, there is a high rate of iron-deficiency anaemia – iron is a mineral obtained mainly from animal sources because, although some vegetables contain it, they contain it in the form of chemical compounds that can't be absorbed in sufficient quantities by our digestive system. More than half the female population of reproductive age is affected by this deficiency [352]. Although diet is not the only cause, it is certainly among the most significant ones.

Clearly, recent bans on the consumption of products of animal origin implemented for political and religious reasons in some provinces will not help correct this problem. In fact, they'll do the reverse and increase the size of the problem [353]. Incidentally, these policies will not improve the welfare of the country's sacred cows, as once they are no longer able to produce milk and they can't be put to any other use, they are abandoned and have to rummage for food in the rubbish, representing a major health risk [354]. This is a clear example that extreme forms of animal rights not only do not improve animal welfare but in fact reduce it.

Malnutrition continues to be one of the four horsemen of the apocalypse. According to the FAO, more than 700 million people (1 in every 10 worldwide) suffers severe malnutrition and up to two billion people have difficulty regularly getting all the nutrients they require. And the COVID pandemic has only exacerbated the problem because both the absolute and relative numbers of people without regular access to food have increased [355].

What about rural populations in less developed countries where these supplements are not available or are too expensive for the general population? How would populations who can only get certain nutrients from animal products deal with this new faith?

The situation is worse for the most defenceless: among children under two years of age, only a third receive the required quantity of food.

The WHO recommends that children of this age consume meat and eggs daily because they are rich in iron and zinc. However, only one in every three children consumes meat or fish daily and only one in five has access to eggs [355].

Why are products of animal origin so important? Firstly because, contrary to what we might think in the West, in much of the world they are the only source of certain nutrients. Large areas between Mongolia and North Africa are arid, so only a few grasses grow. These are regions that, due to their poor soils and extreme climates or because they are mountainous, are not suitable for agriculture. And it is there that animals, especially ruminants, transform these poor-quality grasses into protein and minerals of the highest biological value.

The iron present in foods such as meat is highly absorbable. In contrast, the iron found in vegetables is absorbed in much lower quantities. The same applies for calcium and zinc. Vitamin B_{12}

is not present in plant-sourced food, therefore you have to take supplements of it if you don't eat products of animal origin [355].

Meat contains all the necessary amino acids and provides them in relatively small volumes [356]. Therefore, for example, 6 g of liver provides a child aged 6-23 months with all the vitamins A and B_{12}, folates, calcium, iron and zinc they need a day and with only 9 kilocalories. To provide this same quantity with spinach, we would need 280 g and we would provide 66 kcal [357]. Judge for yourselves which is easier to feed a toddler. The data for adults, and pregnant women in particular, are similar.

Twenty-five grams of liver provides the amount of iron, calcium, zinc, folates, vitamin B_{12} and vitamin A required by an adult person. To obtain these same nutrients from plant products (impossible in the case of vitamin B_{12}) would mean ingesting hundreds of grams.

Both vegans and vegetarians have a lower bone mineral density and that vegans have a higher rate of bone fractures

To give another example: a woman gets her recommended daily intake of iron eating 300 g of beef. To obtain the same amount with lentils and chickpeas, she would need to eat 700 g, or 2.5 kg with spinach. The density of products of animal origin makes them especially important for young children, elderly people, pregnant or breastfeeding women, and people recovering from an illness [358].

It is important to underline that the richness of a food in a certain nutrient is not just quantified by the amount of the nutrient it contains. It is very important that the nutrient can be absorbed in sufficient quantities. For example, 100 g of beef contains 4 mg of iron and 100 g of dried figs contain approximately the same amount. However, once absorbed, we will get 0.7 mg from the meat, but less than 0.2 mg from the figs [359].

Eating nails won't give us enough iron.

We see the same type of difference with other important elements such as zinc or calcium. Zinc is essential for transforming beta-carotene from vegetables (such as carrots) into vitamin A. Insufficient quantities – or absorption – of this mineral makes it more difficult to obtain the necessary amounts of the vitamin.

This deficiency, which is more common in countries with low animal product consumption, has a negative effect on growth, cognitive development and vision, among other things [360].

Regardless of zinc levels, not everyone can efficiently convert beta-carotene (or vitamin A of plant origin) into retinol, which is the form of vitamin A we use [361].

With regard to calcium, a meta-analysis (a study that collected data from almost 500 articles on the subject) concluded that both vegans and vegetarians have a lower bone mineral density and that vegans have a higher rate of bone fractures [362].

The evidence is compelling, and in populations with less access to food of animal origin, this deficiency translates into reduced physical development, and the reverse in populations with more access to such products. This data was obtained from studies performed in more than 100 countries [352] [363].

The children of vegetarian mothers in India show poor development compared to children of mothers whose diet is rich in animal-sourced foods [364].

In countries with low meat and egg consumption, significant iron deficiencies are common among the population, particularly the female population, as we have seen in relation to India. A study conducted in Jordan [365] concluded that, of the 208 patients analysed, 195 had some level of iron-deficiency anaemia. Of these patients, 135 had access to less than 200 g of red meat per week.

It is very dangerous to advocate for these trends as if they are globally applicable, since what is fashionable in the West very quickly becomes a global phenomenon but the consequences are not always the same everywhere.

We might think that this phenomenon is limited to developing countries. However, data shows that a decrease in red meat consumption leads to a significant sections of the population (particularly children, adolescents and women) having a prevalence of this deficiency of more than 10% (it is 5% for men). In some groups, the prevalence was much higher and there was even a significant increase in mortality attributable to the deficiency [366]. In Australia, the data is similar and this deficiency is much more common among vegans and vegetarians [367]. The studies are clear and show that the population that does not eat meat suffers from iron deficiency much more frequently [368].

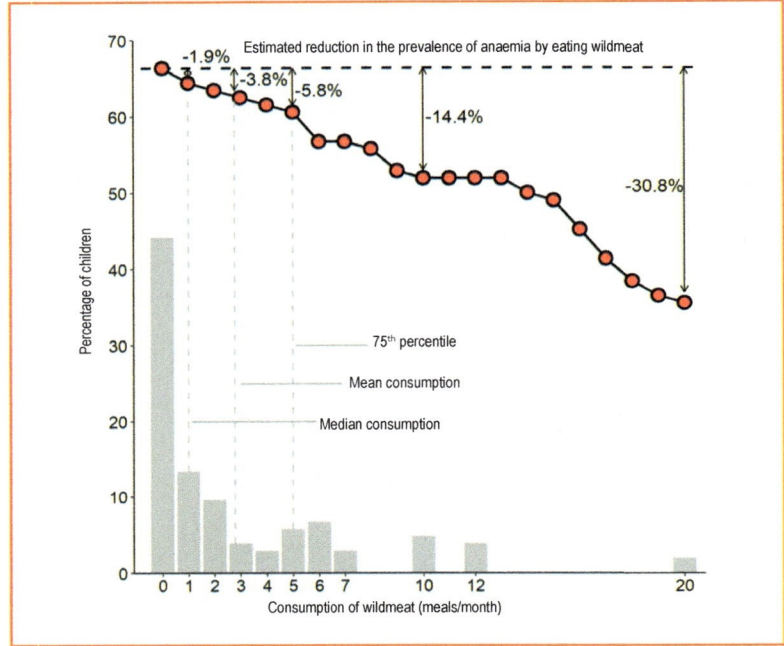

Relationship between the consumption of wildmeat and the prevalence of anaemia among vulnerable children in the central Amazon.

Source: © Nature: Carignano Torres, P., Morsello, C., Orellana, J.D.Y. et al. Wildmeat consumption and child health in Amazonia. Sci Rep 12, 5213 (2022). https://doi.org/10.1038/s41598-022-09260-3

Iron-deficiency anaemia is on the increase in Spain too according to a warning in a recent consensus document published by the Spanish Society of Gynaecology and Obstetrics, which stated that vegetarian diets were the cause of the problem in the country [369] [370].

Another significant aspect is that people who choose to not consume animal products are more prone to depression, anxiety and self-harm. It's not clear whether the absence of certain nutrients induces these behaviours or whether people with a tendency to present these behaviours are more inclined to adopt a vegan diet [371].

Furthermore, in women in particular, muscle mass index is higher in omnivores, even if vegans consume the same quantity of protein of plant origin [372].

Additionally, elderly people with an omnivore diet retain their muscle mass better [373].

I'll finish off this chapter by taking a look at vitamin B_{12}. Among other things, this vitamin is vital for the correct development of our nervous systems, and is only synthesised by certain bacteria in our intestines [374]. However, these microorganisms are at the end of the digestive system and the vitamin they produce must be absorbed in the initial section of the digestive system (in fact, there are animals, such as rodents, that eat their own faeces to obtain this nutrient).

The only exception to this rule are ruminants (cows, sheep and goats), which have stomachs with a high fermentation capacity. In these animals, the bacteria that produce the vitamin are found before the small intestine and, therefore, the animals can absorb it.

Thus, unless we eat our own, or someone else's, faeces, the only way we can get vitamin B_{12} is by consuming products of animal origin because we can only find this nutrient in animal tissue. That's why veganism is a relatively modern movement because, although vegetarianism has existed since antiquity, it was impossible to be vegan due to the lack of artificial vitamin B_{12} supplements, since these supplements are often obtained from genetically modified versions of the bacteria that produce the vitamin [375]. There's no doubt that this process also generates emissions.

In women in particular, muscle mass index is higher in omnivores, even if vegans consume the same quantity of plant protein.

This all demonstrates that not consuming milk, eggs, fish and meat in your diet is possible, but it's not easy. Millions of people cannot afford to do so and millions don't want to. As we have seen, those who opt to do so are a minority, of which a significant proportion go back to omnivore diets. Forcing people to give up animal protein, or even suggesting to people in poor countries – and many in rich countries as well because they also have pockets of poverty – that they should do so, suggesting taxes of up to 30% on meat [376] is not only not sensible, it is morally reprehensible [377] given that, for millions of people, animals represent the only way of accessing vital nutrients and, as we have seen, giving up animal products entails serious risks [378].

Not all products of plant origin are good for your health. It is important to remember that, for example, trans fats, which are mainly of plant origin, are viewed with suspicion and their presence in foods is strictly limited by law due to their harmful effects on health

It is very dangerous to advocate for these trends as if they are globally applicable, since what is fashionable in the West very quickly becomes a global phenomenon but the consequences are not always the same everywhere. Thus, what for us is a good that we can allow ourselves, like organically produced food, in Sri Lanka triggered a crisis of incalculable consequences when the government, following these fashions, banned the use of chemical fertilisers and pesticides, leading the country to ruin and hunger [379]. The same happens when our satiated society gives a distorted vision of the value of animal protein in countries in which meat is a scarce good that is highly necessary and vital for their populations [380].

It is, therefore, scandalous that a scientist who contributed to the creation of a universal, supposedly healthy diet (EAT-Lancet Project) [381] claims that India is the example to follow when it comes to getting proteins from plants [382] when it is, in fact, a country with very high rates of malnutrition.

We shouldn't forget that, when meat is not accessible, a lot of people choose to hunt wild animals, which is a practice that has been associated with the transmission of viruses from animals to humans, as happened with Ebola, AIDS [383] and, possibly, the coronavirus.

MEAT AND CANCER

The suggestion of a link between meat and cancer is another aspect that is often used as a spearhead by vegan publications [384]. Let's see what science has to say on the matter by looking to the institutions that we must all accept as sources of authority.

In this case, we'll use the IARC (International Agency for Research on Cancer), a World Health Organization agency, as a reference.

The IARC creates lists of different substances depending on the confidence, or otherwise, of them being carcinogenic. So, we have [385]:

List 1: Sufficient evidence.

List 2A: Probably carcinogenic (limited evidence).

List 2B: Possibly carcinogenic (there's evidence, but it's not certain)

List 3: No evidence in humans but possibly in experimental animals.

It should be noted – and this is key – that these lists are qualitative and not quantitative [386], i.e., they list substances that can cause cancer, but not the quantity necessary for them to cause cancer. So, sunlight and plutonium are in list 1, but the levels of exposure to the two required to cause cancer are very different.

What does the IARC say about the potential risks of eating meat?

Red meats, according to this agency, are classified in category 2A. Yerba mate (an infusion that's very popular in South America) is also on the list, as is working in a hairdressers' or on a night shift [387]. The evidence of this association between red meat and colorectal cancer is limited and, in fact, the illness is percentage-wise less common in Argentina, a country with a very low consumption, than in Japan, a country with a low very consumption. We shouldn't forget that cancer is a multifactorial disease influenced by elements such as a sedentary lifestyle, smoking and other practices.

For processed meats, the IARC has decided they should be in list 1, with sufficient evidence. However, we have to remember that, in this case, the quantities that can cause cancer are key. According to the IARC itself [388], the daily consumption of 50 g of processed meat results in an absolute increase of 1% in the probability of developing cancer [389] [390] [391].

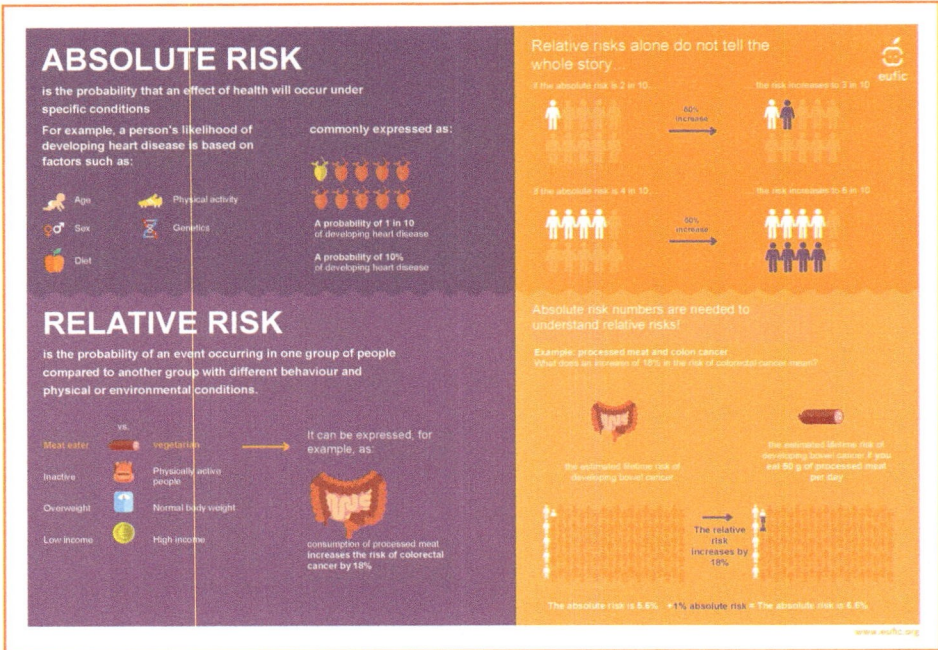

Relative risk vs. absolute risk of eating processed meat. Of every 100 people, 6 will develop colon cancer regardless of their diet.
If they eat 50 g of processed meat every day, 7 out of every 100 will develop the cancer. The relative risk is an increase from 6 to 7, 18% more, but the absolute risk increases from 6% to 7%, i.e. by 1%. It is very important to understand this when reading about the risks of a diet or activity.
Source: The European Food Information Council (EUFIC) www.eufic.org.

As if this data was not enough, other studies published after the IARC lists showed that there are a lot of methodological doubts surrounding data based on observational studies – based on the recollection of what the participants in the studies have eaten in the past – and that it cannot be inferred that meat consumption poses a risk [392]. The media, and even political campaign, triggered by this study was massive [393].

What all the experts do agree on though is that a diet must be varied, rich in nutrients and without excesses. There is no doubt that the Mediterranean diet is a success, some coastal countries have the highest life expectancies of anywhere on earth [394].

However, not all products of plant origin are good for your health. It is important to remember that, for example, trans fats, which are mainly of plant origin, are viewed with suspicion and their presence in foods is strictly limited by law due to their harmful effects on health. In fact, they have been banned in some countries [395] [396].

It is also well known that, after repeated frying, vegetable oils undergo molecular changes that make them potentially harmful to health [397] [398].

No study has been able to demonstrate that vegans or vegetarians live longer or have lower rates of cancer [399] [400].

Opposition to the consumption of meat has always had different motivations and is nothing new or original. Pythagoras, for example, didn't eat it; his reasons included the fact that it caused somnolence [413].

IV

VEGANISM AND RELIGION

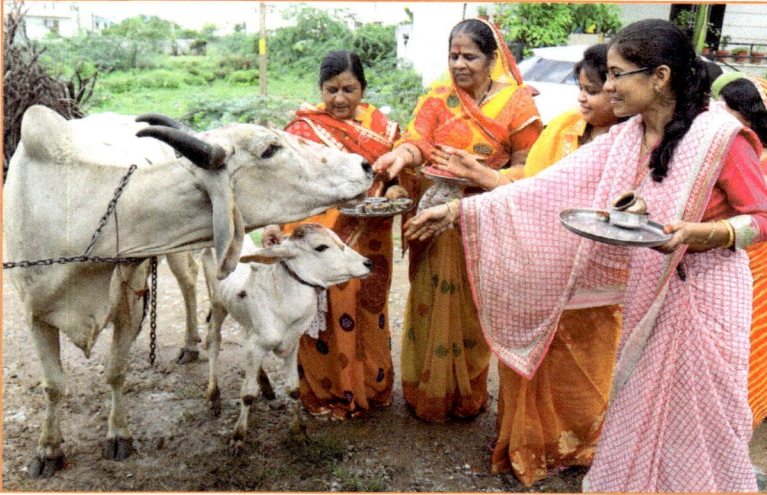

THE SINS OF THE FLESH

Another not insignificant aspect of the reasons, this time religious, for abstinence from meat products is the concern about the relationship between meat consumption and the sins of the flesh. Practically all religious movements limit in some way the consumption of meat, some more explicitly than others and some with greater insistence. And although some, such as Jainism, cite respect for the life of other beings as the main reason (in its most orthodox form, Jains consume only fruit so as not to kill plants), there are more than a few references in their beliefs to the aphrodisiac effects of meat.

Catholicism prohibits the consumption of meat on Fridays during Lent. St. Thomas Aquinas explained that "fasting was instituted by the Church in order to bridle the concupiscences of the flesh..." [402]. The Orthodox Church has a similar approach – although it can be even more restrictive [403]. Other

Christian denominations, such as the adventists, also advocate abstinence from animal products. Some of its pioneers, such as Will Keith Kellogg, encouraged the consumption of cereals at breakfast to replace eggs, bacon and butter. The market for these breakfasts and the brand that he founded have grown exponentially since they first appeared on the scene. Will's brother, John Harvey Kellogg, strongly believed that diet played a key role in inhibiting carnal desires. He believed that cereals and a simple diet acted as anaphrodisiacs, i.e. they decreased libido, and they were recommended as an antidote to onanism [404].

> It turns out that the man who presented himself as the first vegan mayor of the US megacity doesn't say no to a good plate of seafood when given the chance.

Hinduism and Buddhism promote vegetarianism and their reasons also include the unrestrained sexual behaviour that eating meat seems to lead to. Ghandi himself, whose philosophy was based on Jainism and Hinduism, believed in a close link between the consumption of meat and sexuality [405].

The guru Meher Baba also claimed that "the main disadvantage is that eating meat increases sexual desires..." and therefore recommended drinking milk but abstaining from meat, eggs and fish [406].

Hebraic and Islamic faiths are less strict on this issue, although there are some that promote a vegetarian diet [407].

BY WAY OF CONCLUSION

Based on the extensive data provided, we can conclude that a vegan world would be a complete environmental, health and nutritional catastrophe. From a utilitarian perspective, the consequences of a humanity governed by animal rights activists would be devastating for numerous communities as well as for the vast majority of animals.

There is no doubt that everyone should be free to choose how they live and what they eat. We can afford this type of choice in the first world. However, the influence of these ideas on developing countries is very costly for those who live in such countries; we have already seen that low meat consumption in India is one of the causes of anaemia, which is taking on epidemic-like proportions. So, it seems reasonable, setting aside religious considerations, to promote the consumption of meat in the country's population as much as possible and to not present this limitation as the example to follow in terms of diet.

We must, therefore, avoid arbitrary solutions based on conventional wisdom, ideology, prejudices and myths that have no basis other than emotion and the beliefs of those who propagate them.

The domestication of animals was probably the most transcendental qualitative jump and event in all human history. We have been living with them for millennia and much of who we are cannot be understood without animals: nutrition, religious rites, various customs and traditions can only be explained via animals.

No civilisation has been able to do without them. Even today, millions of people live with their animals on farms. They are part of us: for millennia we have eaten their products and they have moulded the landscape in a synergy that benefits both them and us.

Their disappearance would represent a radical change in our society, and a change for the worse, as I have demonstrated in this book.

There is no doubt that the human-animal relationship will continue to evolve. Undoubtedly, there are many aspects of our relationship with them that can be improved and, also undoubtedly, we have evolved by consuming the products they supply us with and the medicines they provide us with. The mutual dependence we have is an equilibrium that we shouldn't be trying to break but rather to improve.

Everyone should be able to choose their preferences, their diet, their values but, on this particular issue, limiting products of animal origin in diets is an arbitrary imposition that isn't supported by any objective data and that would have a very negative impact on the health of some collectives. The absence of animals from our plates or their not pulling a plough in the fields would not improve their welfare (wanting an animal to disappear is not compatible with improving their welfare) nor would it make us more healthy nor improve the environment. Quite the opposite, it would disarm us against numerous diseases which we would lack treatment for, it would incite a lot of populations to hunt wild animals with the associated risk of pandemics, we would lose resources – can you imagine the landscape of Ireland without cows? – and, to round off a list that could be very long, its absence would prevent millions of people from being properly fed and would deprive the third world of the brute strength required to grow crops.

> The absence of animals from our plates or their not pulling a plough in the fields would not improve their welfare nor would it make us more healthy nor improve the environment.

Those last few lines might seem like a slight exaggeration to some readers, since it may seem that there is nothing to prevent us from consuming animal products. However, a magnifying glass allows us to see that some of these limitations are starting to be a concern. We have already commented how getting meat has become almost mission impossible in some provinces of India. But closer to home, in the French city of Lyon, its mayor, an environmentalist, banned meat from school menus and, although he had to row back on his decision a few months later due to protests from parents and students, the intention of some groups is crystal clear [408]. In the Big Apple, state schools have imposed meatless Mondays [409] and a vegan menu every Friday [410]. Taking into account the fact that the majority of pupils come from disadvantaged backgrounds and that school is where many get a square meal every day, it is a huge irresponsibility to put the health of thousands of children at risk for nothing – as we have seen, eliminating all livestock from the USA would reduce greenhouse gas emissions by 2.6%.

But what adds shades of comic opera to these decisions is that the mayor of New York, Eric Adams, himself occasionaly eats fish. It turns out that the man who presented himself as the first vegan mayor of the US megacity won't say no to a good plate of seafood when given the chance [411]. We shouldn't be surprised because, as we have already seen, perseverance is not a strength of vegan diet adopters. Nevertheless, coming from a mayor who forces state school students in his city to give up animal products two days a week, it is an affront, a nonsense and an unacceptable hypocrisy.

Of course, the impact these menus have on the children is much greater than the one they have on the climate since, in addition to their dubious nutritional benefits, children often leave them untouched or simply refuse them, as has been observed in schools in Portland [412].

And, to finish off this point, I want to mention that some countries are seriously considering hefty increases in meat taxes [413]. The intention is to equate this rich source of nutrients with tobacco [414].

It is essential, in the face of so many prejudices and decisions far removed from all scientific evidence, that we are aware of the contributions of both rural animals and the animals that live with us. We must, therefore, avoid arbitrary solutions based on conventional wisdom, ideology, prejudices and myths that have no basis other than emotion and the beliefs of those who propagate them.

Animals, whether pets or farm animals, are indispensable in our society. We owe them respect, a pleasant existence, care and, above all, a greater understanding of their role. Knowing what they offer, which is a lot, and also knowing that between them and us there are insurmountable differences but that these differences do not make them any less worthy of respect, quite the contrary, they should stimulate our curiosity to learn more about them. Only then can we have more consideration and appreciation for what they are and how much they give us.

I hope this book, which is drawing to an end, has contributed to raising awareness of the many contributions they make and that it has helped the reader make decisions based on objective information and data.

BIBLIOGRAPHY

[1]   Diario Veterinario, "Polémica por un libro de texto para niños que desacredita a la ganadería", Diarioveterinario.com, 1 abr. 2021. [*Online*]. Disponible en: https://www.diarioveterinario.com/t/2818772/polemica-libro-texto-ninos-desacredita-ga-naderia.

[2]   YouTube, "'We need to eat the babies' says woman to Alexandria Ocasio-Cortez", 2019. [*Online*]. Disponible en: https://www.youtube.com/watch?v=epwUTVUwB7A.

[3]   Editorial, "¿Quiere salvar el planeta? Coma carne humana", *Catalunya vanguardista*, 23 sep. 2019.

[4]   J. Knopp, "MEATLESS MONDAYS AT SCHOOL: WHY AND HOW SOME SCHOOLS ARE GOING PLANT-BASED", The Human League, 18 jun. 2022. [*Online*]. Disponible en: https://thehumaneleague.org/article/meatless-mondays .

[5]   Tinney, A., "Town pledges to turn vegan-only starting with its schools and hospital", *Metro*, 17 ago. 2022.

[6]   Zelizer, V., *Pricing the Priceless Child*, Princeton: Basic books, 1985.

[7]   Flandrin, J. L., *Le sexe et l'occident*, Paris: Éditions du Seuil, 1981.

[8]   Perfil.com, "Francia: insólito juicio a un gallo denunciado por cantar 'demasiado temprano'", Perfil.com, 7 jun. 2019. [*Online*]. Disponible en: https://www.perfil.com/noticias/internacional/juicio-a-gallo-denunciado-por-cantar-demasiado-tempra-no-en-francia.phtml.

[9]   Illy, B., "Chant du coq ou odeur du fumier : le Parlement adopte une loi pour protéger le 'patrimoine sensoriel' des campagnes", Francetvinfo.fr, 21 ene. 2021. [*Online*]. Disponible en: https://www.francetvinfo.fr/economie/emploi/metiers/droit-et-justice/chant-du-coq-ou-odeur-du-fumier-le-parlement-adopte-une-loi-pour-proteger-le-patrimoine-sensoriel-des-campagnes_4266837.html.

[10]   L'indépendant, "Saint-Ferriol : coq, vaches, clocher… la ruralité c'est ça !", *L'in-dependant*, 15 ene. 2020. [*Online*]. Disponible en: https://www.lindependant.fr/2020/01/15/saint-ferriol-coq-vaches-clocher-la-ruralite-cest-ca,8663939.php.

[11]   La Voz de Asturias, "El cierre de un gallinero se hace viral: 'Un pollo molesta pero el chunda chunda de las terrazas no'", *La Voz de Asturias*, [*Online*]. Disponible en: https://www.lavozdeasturias.es/noticia/viral/2019/05/07/cierre-gallinero-viral-pol-lo-molesta-chunda-chunda-terrazas-/00031557250311773827444.htm.

[12]   Jara y Sedal, "El genial cartel que una ganadera dedica a los urbanitas que visitan su pueblo", Jaraysedal.es, 21 ago. 2021. [*Online*]. Disponible en: https://revistaja-raysedal.es/cartel-ganadera-urbanitas-dedica/.

[13]   PACMA, "El veganismo: una corriente de esperanza para el planeta", Disponible en: https://pacma.es/el-veganismo-una-corriente-de-esperanza-para-el-planeta/, 2018.

[14]   ADDA, "Manifiesto programático de la Asociación Defensa Derechos Animal, ADDA, que necesariamente asumen sus Socios y Miembros Colaboradores", https://www.addaong.org/es/quienes-somos/manifiesto/, 2018.

[15]   Corroto, P., "La hora del manifiesto animalista", *El País*, Disponible en: https://el-pais.com/cultura/2018/01/28/actualidad/1517162827_605464.html, 28 Enero 2018.

[16]   PETA, "Peta.org", Peta, 2021. [*Online*]. Disponible en: https://www.peta.org/.

[17]   Steiner, G., "Animal, Vegetal, Miserable", *The New York Times*, 22 nov. 2009.

[18]   Climatedepot, "Former UN Climate Chief: Meat eaters should be banished, treated 'the same way that smokers are treated'", *Climate depot,* Disponible en: https://www.climatedepot.com/2018/12/07/former-un-climate-chief-meat-eaters-should-be-banished-treated-the-same-way-that-smokers-are-treated/, 7 dic. 2018.

[19]   Party for the Animals, [*Online*]. Disponible en: https://www.partyfortheanimals.com/es/quienes-somos?lang=es.

[20]   Party for the Animals, [*Online*]. Disponible en: https://www.partyfortheanimals.com/en/documentation/our-videos.

[21]   N. G. P. Foundation, "Documentary Meat the Truth", [*Online*]. Disponible en: https://www.ngpf.nl/en/documentary-meat-the-truth/.

[22]   Novella, S., "PETA Embraces Autism Pseudoscience", Science Based Medicine, 28 may. 2014. [*Online*]. Disponible en: https://sciencebasedmedicine.org/peta-embraces-autism-pseudoscience/.

[23]   Veggiepride, "Veggiepride.org", [*Online*]. Disponible en: http://www.veggiepride.org/.

[24]   Pelluchon, C., "La cause animale aujourd'hui - Veggie Pride 2017", YouTube, 6 Oct 2017. [*Online*]. Disponible en: https://www.youtube.com/watch?v=p0W2ACNwb7Y. [Acceso 2 mar 2021].

[25]   Rodríguez, J. y Mateos, A., *La dieta que nos hizo humanos*, Junta de Castilla y León, 2011.

[26]   Zink, K., "Impact of meat and Lower Palaeolithic food processing techniques on chewing in humans", *Nature* 531, pp. 500-503, 2016.

[27]   Faunalytics, "A Summary Of Faunalytics' Study Of Current And Former Vegetarians And Vegans", Faunalytics, 24 feb. 2016. [*Online*]. Disponible en: https://faunalytics.org/a-summary-of-faunalytics-study-of-current-and-former-vegetarians-and-vegans/#.

[28]   Herzog, H., "84% of Vegetarians and Vegans Return to Meat. Why?", *Psycology Today,* 2 dic. 2014.

[29]   Herzog, H., "Why do most vegetarians go back to eating meat", *Psycology today,* Disponible en: https://www.psychologytoday.com/gb/blog/animals-and-us/201106/why-do-most-vegetarians-go-back-eating-meat, 20 June 2011.

[30]   Keith, L., *The Vegetarian Myth*, Crescent City: Flashpoint press, 2009.

[31]   Schultz, C., "Most Vegetarians Lapse After Only a Year", *Smithsonian magazine,* Disponible en: https://www.smithsonianmag.com/smart-news/most-vegetarians-lapse-after-only-year-180953565/?no-ist, 2014.

[32]   DeSantis, R., "Vegan YouTuber Apologizes After She's Caught Eating Fish: 'I Made a Mistake'", *People,* Disponible en: https://people.com/food/vegan-youtuber-rawvana-apologizes-caught-eating-fish/, 20 mar. 2019.

[33]   Smith, E., "Inside the 'secret' meat menu at exalted 'vegan' spot Eleven Madison Park", Page Six, 29 sep. 2021. [*Online*]. Disponible en: https://pagesix.com/2021/09/29/vegan-eleven-madison-park-offers-secret-meat-menu-for-the-rich/.

[34]   Chumley, C. K., "Bill Clinton falls off vegan diet wagon - but not vegan label", *Washington times,* Disponible en: https://www.washingtontimes.com/news/2014/apr/15/bill-clinton-falls-vegan-diet-wagon-not-vegan-labe/, 15 abr. 2014.

[35]   Agrimer, "Végétariens et Flexitariens En France en 2020", France Agrimer, París, 2021.

[36]   Stahler, C., "How Many People Are Vegan?", *The vegetarian resource group,* Disponible en: https://www.vrg.org/nutshell/Polls/2019_adults_veg.htm, 2019.

[37]   Peter, O., "Number Of Vegans in UK Soars To 3.5 Million, Survey Finds", *The Independent,* Disponible en: https://www.independent.co.uk/life-style/food-and-drink/vegans-uk-rise-popularity-plant-based-diets-veganism-figures-survey-compare-market-a8286471.html, 5 abr. 2018.

[38]   National Statistics, "Food Statistics in your pocket: Global and UK supply", National Statistics, 30 nov. 2020. [*Online*]. Disponible en: https://www.gov.uk/government/statistics/food-statistics-pocketbook/food-statistics-in-your-pocket-global-and-uk-supply.

[39]   Yoder, K., "'I had a meatmare': Why flesh haunts the dreams of vegetarians", Grist, 13 jun. 2017. [*Online*]. Disponible en: https://grist.org/article/i-had-a-meatmare-why-flesh-haunts-the-dreams-of-vegetarians/.

[40]   OPP, "Grants", Disponible en: https://www.openphilanthropy.org/giving/grants, 2020, 2017.

[41]   Katasi, S., "The Truth About The Guardian's Plant-Based 'Ethics'", *AdaptNation*, Disponible en: https://adapnation.io/theguardian-plantbased-ethics/, 3 jul. 2020.

[42]   Luneau, G., *Steak Barbare*, Éditions de l'Aube, 2020.

[43]   McMorris, B., "My Vegan Hell", The Spectator, 13 feb. 2020. [*Online*]. Disponible en: https://spectator.us/life/vegan-hell-bill-mcmorris/. [Acceso 13 mar. 2021].

[44]   Clerx, A., "Is Veganism a Religion?", *European Academy on Religion and Society*, Disponible en: https://europeanacademyofreligionandsociety.com/news/is-veganism-a-religion/, 27 may. 2020.

[45]   Wright, P., "Be Careful What You Dismiss as Not a 'Real' Religion When Employees Seek Religious Accommodation: Court Holds Veganism Could Plausibly Be a 'Religious Belief'", *Employer Law Report*, Disponible en: https://www.employerlawreport.com/2013/01/articles/eeo/be-careful-what-you-dismiss-as-not-a-real-religion-when-employees-seek-religious-accommodation-court-holds-veganism-could-plausibly-be-a-religious-belief/, 8 ene. 2013.

[46]   "Is My Phone Powered By Child Labour?", Amnesty International, 2016. [*Online*]. Disponible en: https://www.amnesty.org/en/latest/campaigns/2016/06/drc-cobalt-child-labour/.

[47]   Jackson Njehia, N. M., "Elephants or avocados: a Kenyan dilemma", Reuters, 3 mar. 2021. [*Online*]. Disponible en: https://www.reuters.com/article/us-kenya-environment-elephants/elephants-or-avocados-a-kenyan-dilemma-idUSKBN2AV10L.

[48]   Horn, R., "Monkey slavery: Is your coconut milk really vegan?", The Vegan Review, 19 ago. 2020. [*Online*]. Disponible en: https://theveganreview.com/monkey-slavery-is-your-coconut-milk-really-vegan/.

[49]   "La tortura experimental", Vegetarianismo.net, [*Online*]. Disponible en: https://vegetarianismo.net/liberacionanimal/salt-experimentacion.html.

[50]   PETA, "Is SeaWorld Bad? Check Out These Shocking Marine Park Facts", PETA, 27 ene. 2020. [*Online*]. Disponible en: https://www.seaworldofhurt.com/features/is-seaworld-bad-animal-abuse-cruelty-facts/.

[51]   "Los zoos son cárceles de animales", Una familia vegana y normal, 4 jun. 2020. [*Online*]. Disponible en: https://unafamiliaveganaynormal.com/los-zoos-son-carceles-de-animales/.

[52]   Barrio, A. d., "Los taurinos anuncian querellas contra los tuiteros que se mofan de la muerte de Víctor Barrio", *El Mundo*, 11 jul. 2016. [*Online*]. Disponible en: https://www.elmundo.es/cultura/2016/07/11/5783788f268e3ebe738b456c.html.

[53]   Abraham, E., "Abuse, intimidation, death threats: the vicious backlash facing former vegans", *The Guardian*, 4 dic. 2021. [*Online*]. Disponible en: https://www.theguardian.com/lifeandstyle/2021/dec/04/abuse-intimidation-death-threats-the-vicious-backlash-facing-fomer-vegans?CMP=twt_a-environment_b-gdneco.

[54]   Young, P., "The blueprint. Fur Industry Analysis. Weak Links. Addresses. A complete guide to end the fur industry", Warcry communications, Disponible en: https://www.coalitionagainstfurfarms.com/wp-content/uploads/2020/01/Blueprint-2020-Fur-Farm-List.pdf, 2020.

[55]   Wikipedia, "Frente de Liberación Animal", Wikipedia, [*Online*]. Disponible en: https://es.wikipedia.org/wiki/Frente_de_Liberaci%C3%B3n_Animal.

[56]   Bite back, "News from the Frontlines", Bite back, 2021. [*Online*]. Disponible en: https://www.directaction.info/news.htm.

[57] Wikipedia, "Steven Best", Wikipedia, [*Online*]. Disponible en: https://en.wikipedia.org/wiki/Steven_Best.

[58] Poingt, G., "'Il se sentait seul et isolé' : pourquoi 600 agriculteurs se suicident chaque année ?", *Le Figaro*, 1 12 2020. [*Online*]. Disponible en: https://www.lefigaro.fr/social/il-se-sentait-seul-et-isole-pourquoi-600-agriculteurs-se-suicident-chaque-annee-20201201.

[59] Campion, E., "Pourquoi un agriculteur se suicide tous les deux jours en France?", *Le Figaro*, 17 ago. 2018. [*Online*]. Disponible en: https://www.lefigaro.fr/vox/societe/2018/08/17/31003-20180817ARTFIG00252-pourquoi-un-agriculteur-se-suicide-t-il-tous-les-deux-jours-en-france.php.

[60] McMahan, J., "The problem of predation", in *Philosophy comes to dinner*, New York, Routledge, 2016, pp. 268-295.

[61] Sagoff, M., "Animal Liberation and Environmental Ethics: Bad Marriage, Quick Divorce", *Osgoode Hall Law Journal*, vol. 22, n.° 2, pp. 297-307, 1984.

[62] Bittel, J., "Seagulls Have a Gruesome New Way of Attacking Baby Seals", *National Geographic*, 17 ago. 2015. [*Online*]. Disponible en: https://www.nationalgeographic.com/news/2015/08/150817-seals-seagulls-animals-science-predators-prey/#:~:text=Kelp%20gulls%20are%20eating%20the,nature%2C%20a%20new%20study%20says.&text=Seagulls%20have%20developed%20a%20hunting,pups%2C%20a%20new%20study%20.

[63] YouTube, [*Online*]. Disponible en: https://www.youtube.com/watch?v=_yAi8KrvHa4.

[64] Smith, D., "Wolf pup survival a fragile thing", *Star Tribune*, 5 mar. 2015. [*Online*]. Disponible en: https://www.startribune.com/wolf-pup-survival-a-fragile-thing/295226071/.

[65] "Lion vs Hippo Lion's Jaw is Breaking Off", YouTube, [*Online*]. Disponible en: https://www.youtube.com/watch?v=LtE0N43_t3A.

[66] "HORROR. Wild dogs eat live warthog", YouTube, [*Online*]. Disponible en: https://www.youtube.com/watch?v=J8PfuWaJ6bQ.

[67] "Graphic content warning: Baboon eats gazelle alive", Daily motion, [*Online*]. Disponible en: https://www.dailymotion.com/video/xsd0ta.

[68] La-Philo, "La Philosophie Des Lumières", La-Philo, [*Online*]. Disponible en: https://la-philosophie.com/philosophie-lumieres.

[69] Wilcox, C., "Bambi or Bessie: Are wild animals happier?", Scientific American Guest Blog, 11 abr. 2011. [*Online*]. Disponible en: https://blogs.scientificamerican.com/guest-blog/bambi-or-bessie-are-wild-animals-happier/.

[70] E. Britannica, "Silkworm moth", 21 may. 2020. [*Online*]. Disponible en: https://www.britannica.com/animal/silkworm-moth. [Acceso 25 abr. 2021].

[71] Chansigaud, V., *Histoire de la Domestication*, Paris: Delachaux et Niestlé, 2020.

[72] Darwin, C., *The Variation of Animals and Plants under Domestication*, John Murray, 1868.

[73] D. 2008/120/CE, *DIRECTIVA 2008/120/CE*, 2009.

[74] Ministerio de Agricultura, "Noticias del exterior 472", Ministerio de Agricultura, Pesca y Alimentación, Madrid, 2021.

[75] Manteca, X., *Bienestar animal*, Barcelona : Gráfica IN Multimédica, 2020.

[76] Wikipedia, [*Online*]. Disponible en: https://en.wikipedia.org/wiki/Compassion_in_World_Farming.

[77] C. i. a. farming, "End the cage age", [*Online*]. Disponible en: https://www.endthecageage.eu/#ourCampaign.

[78] Appleby, M. y Cooper, J., "Demand for nest boxes in laying hens", *Behavioural Processes*, vol. 36, pp. 171-182, 1996.

[79] Hales, J., "Higher preweaning mortality in free farrowing pens compared with farrowing crates in three commercial pig farms", *The Animal Consortium*, pp. 113-120, 2014.

[80]   "Gal Association", [Online]. Disponible en: https://www.globalanimallaw.org/patron-age/global/donald-broom.html.

[81]   Thorpe, W., "The assessment of pain and distress in animals", Her Majesty Stationery Office, London, 1965.

[82]   Lusk, J., Compassion by the pound, Oxford University Press, 2011.

[83]   Spoolder, H. et al., "Initiatives to reduce mutilations in EU livestock production", Wageningen University, The Netherlands, Wageningen, 2016.

[84]   Turner, S. y Dwyer, C., "Welfare Assessment in Extensive Animal Production Systems: Challenges and Opportunities", Animal Welfare, vol. 16, pp. 189-192, 2007.

[85]   Berckmans, D., "Precision livestock farming technologies for welfare management in intensive livestock systems", Rev Sci Tech, vol. 33, n.º 1, pp. 189-196, 2014.

[86]   Lyles, J. L. y Calvo-Lorenzo, M., "Practical developments in managing animal welfare in beef cattle: What does the future hold?", Journal of Animal Science, vol. 92, n.º 12, pp. 5334-5344, 2014.

[87]   Beek, V., "ASF Germany: Free-range farm depopulated; case in Frankfurt/Oder", Pig Progress, 4 mar. 2021. [Online]. Disponible en: https://www.pigprogress.net/Health/Articles/2021/3/ASF-Germany-Free-range-farm-depopulated-case-in-FrankfurtOder-717781E/.

[88]   "Ethiopian Great Famine – 1888-1892", Devastating Disasters, [Online]. Disponible en: https://devastatingdisasters.com/ethiopian-great-famine-1888-1892/.

[89]   Amanda, K. M., The Rinderpest Campaigns, Cambridge University Press, 2018.

[90]   Animal Health,"Arranca el proyecto VACDIVA, una vacuna contra la peste porcina africana", Animal's Health, 18 nov. 2019. [Online]. Disponible en: https://www.animalshealth.es/profesionales/arranca-el-proyecto-vacdiva-de-vacuna-contra-la-peste-porcina-africana-ppa-dirigido-por-sanchez-vizcaino.

[91]   Arredondo, A. et al., "Enfermedad hemorrágica del conejo", Boletín de cunicultura, n.º 193, pp. 22-25.

[92]   Animal Health, "Un proyecto contra la enfermedad hemorrágica del conejo en el Mediterráneo", Animals Health, 15 oct. 2020. [Online]. Disponible en: https://www.animalshealth.es/profesionales/proyecto-enfermedad-hemorragica-conejo-mediter-raneo.

[93]   FAO, "The State of World Fisheries and Aquaculture 2020. Sustainability in action. Rome", FAO, Rome, 2020.

[94]   Compassion in World Farming, "Is The Next Pandemy On Our Plates?", 2020.

[95]   Terregino C. et al., "Active surveillance for avian influenza viruses in wild birds and backyard flocks in Northern Italy during 2004 to 2006", Avian Pathology, vol. 36, n.º 4, pp. 337-4, 2007.

[96]   ECDC, "Avian influenza overview February", European Centre for Disease Prevention and Control, 2021.

[97]   Ministerio de Agricultura, "Manual práctico de operaciones en la lucha contra la influenza aviar", oct. 2019. [Online]. Disponible en: https://www.mapa.gob.es/es/ganaderia/temas/sanidad-animal-higiene-ganadera/manualiaoctubre2019_tcm30-437988.pdf.

[98]   Avert, "Origin of HIV & AIDS", Avert, 30 oct. 2019. [Online]. Disponible en: https://www.avert.org/professionals/history-hiv-aids/origin.

[99]   WHO, "Ebola virus disease", WHO, 23 mar. 2021. [Online].

[100]   Pascual, J., "¿Por qué las vacunas deben su nombre a las vacas?", Naukas.com, 28 ene. 2017. [Online]. Disponible en: https://naukas.com/2017/01/28/por-que-las-vacunas-deben-su-nombre-a-las-vacas/.

[101]   Anderson, J., "Going Vegan Or Vegetarian: Motivations & Influences", Faunalytics, 8 dic. 2021. [Online]. Disponible en: https://faunalytics.org/going-veg-motivations-and-influences/.

[102]   Carson, B., "Sex, lies, and eggless mayonnaise: Something is rotten at food startup Hampton Creek, former employees say", Insider, 6 ago. 2015. [Online]. Disponible en: https://www.businessinsider.com/hampton-creek-ceo-complaints-2015-7?IR=T.

[103]   Summer, J. V., "Should Vegans Eat Roadkill?", *Tenderly*, Disponible en: https://me-dium.com/tenderlymag/should-vegans-eat-roadkill-8765b95f62f3, 26 Feb 2020.

[104]   Bruckner, D. W., "Strict Vegetarianism Is Immoral", in *The Moral Complexities of Eating Meat*, New York, Oxford University Press, 2016, pp. 30-47.

[105]   Agnew, S., "Can vegans and vegetarians consume their placenta?", Placenta Rem-edies Network, 12 abr. 2018. [*Online*]. Disponible en: https://placentaremediesnet-work.org/can-vegans-and-vegetarians-consume-their-placenta/.

[106]   Bunton, S., "11 Celebrities Who Ate Their Placenta & Are Happy To Admit It", Romper, 6 jul. 2016. [*Online*]. Disponible en: https://www.romper.com/p/11-celebri-ties-who-ate-their-placenta-are-happy-to-admit-it-13659.

[107]   Satya, "Singer Says The Satya Interview with Peter Singer", Satyamag.com, oct. 2006. [*Online*]. Disponible en: http://www.satyamag.com/oct06/singer.html.

[108]   Archer, M., "Ordering the vegetarian meal? There's more animal blood on your hands", *The Conversation*, 15 dic. 2011.

[109]   Tew, T. y Macdonald, D., "The effects of harvest on arable wood mice Apodemus sylvaticus,", *Biological Conservation*, vol. 65, n.° 3, pp. 279-283, 1993.

[110]   Davis, S. L., "THE LEAST HARM PRINCIPLE MAY REQUIRE THAT HUMANS CON-SUME A DIET CONTAINING LARGE HERBIVORES, NOT A VEGAN DIET", *Journal of Agricultural and Environmental Ethics 16*, pp. 387-394, 2003.

[111]   Fisher B. y Lamey, A., "Field Deaths in Plant Agriculture", *Journal of Agricultural and Environmental Ethics 31*, pp. 409-428, 2018.

[112]   "Ordering the vegetarian meal? There's more animal blood on your hands", The Conversation, 15 dic. 2011. [*Online*]. Disponible en: https://theconversation.com/ordering-the-vegetarian-meal-theres-more-animal-blood-on-your-hands-4659.

[113]   Tomasik, B., "Crop Cultivation and Wild Animals", reducing-suffering.org, 22 may. 2019. [*Online*]. Disponible en: https://reducing-suffering.org/crop-cultiva-tion-and-wild-animals/#Killing_vertebrates_during_harvesting.

[114]   M. Evans, "So you're a vegan ... but are you, really?", *The Australian*, 29 jun. 2019.

[115]   Needham, K., "200,000 native ducks shot as pests of rice crops", The Sydney Morn-ing Herald, 3 Aug 2014. [*Online*]. Disponible en: https://www.smh.com.au/national/nsw/200000-native-ducks-shot-as-pests-of-rice-crops-20140802-zzrjj.html.

[116]   "En peligro de muerte 100.000 pájaros por la recogida nocturna de aceituna", *La Voz de Almería*, no. En peligro de muerte 100.000 pájaros por la recogida nocturna de aceituna, Disponible en: https://www.lavozdealmeria.com/noticia/3/provin-cia/162940/en-peligro-de-muerte-100-000-pajaros-por-la-recogida-nocturna-de-aceituna, 29 nov. 2018.

[117]   Eplett, L., "Rub a Dub Dub, Is It Time to Eat Grubs?", *Scientific American Blog*, Disponible en: https://blogs.scientificamerican.com/guest-blog/grubs-as-grub/, 4 jun. 2013.

[118]   Mundovegano, "Por qué los veganos no tomamos miel", *Mundo Vegano*, Dis-ponible en: https://mundovegano.org/por-que-los-veganos-no-tomamos-miel/, 14 ene. 2018.

[119]   Code rural et de la pêche maritime : *Titre II : Mesures de prévention, surveil-lan ... (Articles L221-1 à L228-8)*. Disponible en: https://www.legifrance.gouv.fr/codes/section_lc/LEGITEXT000006071367/LEGISCTA000006138322/#LEGISC-TA000024396682

[120]   BBC News, "Coronavirus: Dinamarca sacrificará 17 millones de visones por una 'riesgosa' mutación de covid-19", BBC News, 5 nov. 2020. [*Online*]. Disponible en: https://www.bbc.com/mundo/noticias-54824991.

[121]   PETA, "Living in Harmony with Rats", Disponible en: https://www.peta.org/issues/wildlife/living-harmony-wildlife/rats/, 28 oct. 2020.

[122]   Singer, P., *Practical Ethics*, Cambridge University Press, 1999.

[123]   Kant, E., *Lecciones de ética*, Barcelona: Crítica, 1988.

[124]   Regan, T., *The Case for Animal Rights*, Berkeley: University of California Press, 2004.

[125]   Regan, T., *Defending Animal Rights*, University of Illinois Press, 2001.

[126]   Dawkins, M. S., *Why Animals Matter*, Oxford University Press, 2021.

[127]   Regan, T., "The Other Victim", The Hasting Center Report, 1985.

[128]   Singer, P., *Animal Liberation*, p. 22: Avon Books, 1975.

[129]   Dimmock, M. y Fisher, A., *Ethics for A Level*, Cambridge: Open Book Publisher, 2017.

[130]   Singer, P., "Peter Singer", 2020. [*Online*]. Disponible en: https://petersinger.info/faq/.

[131]   McLean, A., *The Elimination of Morality*, New York: Routledge, 1993.

[132]   Regan, T., "YouTube", [*Online*]. Disponible en: https://www.youtube.com/watch?v=aEJBp-GXmqA.

[133]   Martin, M., "A Critique of Moral Vegetarianism", *Reason papers 3*, pp. 13-43, 1976.

[134]   Wikipedia, "Richard D. Ryder", Wikipedia, 6 ago. 2021. [*Online*]. Disponible en: https://en.wikipedia.org/wiki/Richard_D._Ryder.

[135]   Wells, T., "The Incoherence of Peter Singer's Utilitarian Argument for Vegetarianism", ABC Religion & Ethics, 24 oct. 2016. [*Online*]. Disponible en: https://www.abc.net.au/religion/the-incoherence-of-peter-singers-utilitarian-argument-for-vegeta/10096418.

[136]   Pauer-Studer, H., "Peter Singer on Euthanasia", *The Monist*, vol. 76, n.° 2, pp. 135-157, 1993.

[137]   "Un miracle assez effrayant" : un père de famille sort du coma après avoir été débranché
Disponible en: https://www.tf1info.fr/international/etats-unis-scott-marr-un-pere-de-famille-du-nebraska-se-reveille-de-son-coma-apres-avoir-ete-debranche-2109385.html

[138]   Lee, P. y George, R., "Chapter 16: The Nature and Basis of Human Dignity (The President's Council on Bioethics)", Bioethics archive, Washington DC, 2008.

[139]   Carruthers, P., *The animals issue*, Cambridge University Press, 1994.

[140]   Singer, P., "Animal Liberation", New York, Avon books, 1977, pp. 178-179.

[141]   Wikipedia. [*Online*]. Disponible en: https://en.wikipedia.org/wiki/Congenital_insensitivity_to_pain.

[142]   Savater, F., "Regueifas de Ciencia'16: ¿Está justificado el uso de animales en experimentación científica?", YouTube, [*Online*]. Disponible en: https://www.youtube.com/watch?v=M2O-ku7alJw.

[143]   Wei-Haas, M., "You may have more Neanderthal DNA than you think", *National Geographic*, 30 ene. 2020. [*Online*]. Disponible en: https://www.nationalgeographic.com/science/article/more-neanderthal-dna-than-you-think.

[144]   Sodesaki, K., "The legal status of a human corpse", *Nihon Hoigaku Zasshi*, vol. 55, n.° 2, pp. 235-242, 2001.

[145]   Hammack, C. M., *The Law And Ethics Of Using The Dead In Research*, Winston-Salem, North Carolina, 2014.

[146]   Lithwick, D., "Habeas Corpses", Slate, 14 Mar 2002. [*Online*]. Disponible en: https://slate.com/news-and-politics/2002/03/what-are-the-rights-of-dead-people.html.

[147]   Molia, M., "Por qué es injustificable exhibir cadáveres humanos", *La Vanguardia*, 14 jun. 2021.

[148]   Le Figaro, "Paris-Descartes : l'ancien président de l'université mis en examen pour «atteinte à l'intégrité d'un cadavre", *Le Figaro*, 7 jul. 2021.

[149]   Le Figaro Rédaction, "Viols d'une centaine de cadavres à l'hôpital : le scandale qui secoue le Royaume-Uni", *Le Figaro*, 8 nov. 2021. [*Online*]. Disponible en: https://www.lefigaro.fr/flash-actu/agressions-sexuelles-post-mortem-au-royaume-uni-une-enquete-independante-ouverte-20211108.

[150]   Gleeson, A., "Eating Meat and Reading Diamond", *Philosophical papers*, vol. 37, n.° 1, pp. 157-175, 2008.

[151]   Diamond, C., "Eating Meat and Eating People", *Philosophy*, vol. 53, n.° 206, pp. 465-479, 1978.

[152]   Hsiao, T., "In Defense of Eating Meat", *Agric Environ Ethics*, vol. 28, pp. 277-291, 2015.

[153]   ISE, "Peter Singer and Eugenics", Institute for Social Ecology, 2009. [*Online*]. Disponible en: https://social-ecology.org/wp/2005/01/peter-singer-and-eugenics/.

[154]   Singer, P., "A German Attack on Applied Ethics. A Statement by Peter Singer", *Journal of Applied Philosophy*, vol. 9, n.° 1, 1992.

[155]   Johnson, H. M., "Unspeakable Conversations", *The New York Times Magazine*, 2003.

[156]   Dynamics, L., "Peter Singer Doesn't Want Tax Dollars to Pay for Disabled Babies", Life Dynamics, 30 jun. 2015. [*Online*]. Disponible en: https://blog.lifedynamics.com/peter-singer-doesnt-want-tax-dollars-pay-disabled-babies/.

[157]   Oderberg, D., "Why Peter Singer is wrong", YouTube, 30 oct. 2017. [*Online*]. Disponible en: https://www.youtube.com/watch?v=Wfc4uS3HBSw.

[158]   Krantz, S. L., *Refuting Peter Singer's Ethical Theory*, Westport: Praeger Publishers, 2002.

[159]   Singer, P., "About me", Peter Singer, [*Online*]. Disponible en: https://petersinger.info/about-me-cv.

[160]   Slate, "The Bestiality Perplex", Slate, 2 abr. 2001. [*Online*]. Disponible en: https://slate.com/news-and-politics/2001/04/the-bestiality-perplex.html.

[161]   Olasky, M., "Peter Singer, bestiality, and infanticide", Thinking to Believe, 8 may. 2009. [*Online*]. Disponible en: https://thinkingtobelieve.com/2009/05/08/peter-singer-bestiality-and-infanticide/.

[162]   Pool, C., "Princeton University professor says, sex with dogs is harmless: 'I know women who say it pleases them.'", Caldron pool, 18 ago. 2018. [*Online*]. Disponible en: https://caldronpool.com/princeton-university-professor-says-sex-with-dogs-is-harmless-i-know-women-who-say-it-pleases-them/.

[163]   Robinson, N. J., "Now Peter Singer Argues That It Might Be Okay To Rape Disabled People", Current Affairs, 4 abr. 2017. [*Online*]. Disponible en: https://www.currentaffairs.org/2017/04/now-peter-singer-argues-that-it-might-be-okay-to-rape-disabled-people.

[164]   Frey, R. G., *Interests and Rights. The case against animals*, Oxford University Press, 1980.

[165]   Mancuso, S. y Viola, A., *Brilliant Green*, Island Press, 2015.

[166]   ECNH, "The Dignity of Living Beings With Regards To Plants", Ariane Willemsen, ECNH Secretariat, Berne, 2008.

[167]   Phys.org, "Scientists teach worms to learn", Phys.org, 11 nov. 2005. [*Online*]. Disponible en: https://phys.org/news/2005-11-scientists-worms.html.

[168]   Gershman, S. J., "Reconsidering the evidence for learning in Single Cells", *eLife*, 2021.

[169]   Robots.net, "Who Is Sophia the Robot: Everything You Need to Know About Her", Robots.net, 8 July 2020. [*Online*]. Disponible en: https://robots.net/ai/who-is-sophia-the-robot-everything-you-need-to-know-about-her/.

[170]   ASPCR, "ASPCR.com", American Society for the Preventio of Cruelty to Robots, 2016. [*Online*]. Disponible en: http://www.aspcr.com/index.html.

[171]   Sigfusson, L., "Do Robots Deserve Human Rights?", Discovermagazine.com, 5 dic. 2017. [*Online*]. Disponible en: https://www.discovermagazine.com/technology/do-robots-deserve-human-rights.

[172]   N. Heller, "If Animals Have Rights, Should Robots?", The New Yorker, 20 nov. 2016. [*Online*]. Disponible en: https://www.newyorker.com/magazine/2016/11/28/if-animals-have-rights-should-robots.

[173]   Jiang, L., "Towards Machine Ethics and Norms", AI2 blog, 4 nov. 2021. [*Online*]. Disponible en: https://blog.allenai.org/towards-machine-ethics-and-norms-d64f2bd-de6a3?gi=6cfdaf3eea8e.

[174]   Ferràs, X., "La conquista de la consciencia", *La Vanguardia*, 26 jun. 2022.

[175]   Ramachandran, V. S., *Phantoms in the Brain*, Harper Perennial, 1999.

[176]   Wikipedia, "Miembro fantasma", Wikipedia, [*Online*]. Disponible en: https://es-.wikipedia.org/wiki/Miembro_fantasma.

[177]   Ramachadran, V. S. , "Vilayanur Ramachadran habla sobre sus mentes", Ted Talk, [*Online*]. Disponible en: https://www.youtube.com/watch?v=Rl2LwnaUA-k.

[178]   IASP, "PAIN", IASP, 2021. [*Online*]. Disponible en: https://www.iasp-pain.org/publications/pain/.

[179]   N. R. C., *Recognition and Alleviation of Pain in Laboratory Animals*, Washington (DC): National Academies Press, 2009.

[180]   Crook, R. y Walters, E., "Nociceptive Behavior and Physiology of Molluscs: Animal Welfare Implications", *ILAR Journal*, vol. 52, n.° 2, pp. 185-195, 2019.

[181]   Riordan, H., "26 Gunshot Survivors Explain Exactly What The Bullet Felt Like", Thought Catalogue, 6 Feb 2017. [*Online*]. Disponible en: https://thoughtcatalog.com/holly-riordan/2017/02/26-gunshot-survivors-explain-exactly-what-the-bullet-felt-like/.

[182]   Smith E. St. *et al.*, "Independent evolution of pain insensitivity in African mole-rats: origins and mechanisms", *J Comp Physiol A Neuroethol Sens Neural Behav Physiol.* , vol. 206, n.° 3, pp. 313-325, 2020.

[183]   Eisemann, C. H. *et al.*, "Do insects feel pain? — A biological view", *Experientia*, vol. 40, pp. 164-167 , 1984.

[184]   J. D. R. *et al.*, *Fish and Fisheries*, Blackwell Publishing, 2012.

[185]   Wolff, F., *Notre humanité. D'Aristote aux neurosciences*, Librarie Arthème Fayard, 2010.

[186]   YouTube, "Homme et Animal : une limite arbitraire - Corine Pelluchon", YouTube, [*Online*]. Disponible en: https://www.youtube.com/watch?v=cGUc3ktflcM.

[187]   Campillo, S., "Qué son las personas no humanas?", Hipertextual, 23 Feb 2016. [*Online*]. Disponible en: https://hipertextual.com/2016/02/personas-no-humanas.

[188]   Bimbenet, É., *Le complexe des trois singes*, Paris: Éditions du Seuil, 2017.

[189]   Carbonell, E. *et al.*, "*Homo sapiens*: ¿quiénes somos?", *Mètode*, 27 sep. 2017. [*Online*]. Disponible en: https://metode.es/revistas-metode/monograficos/homo-sapiens-quienes-somos.html.

[190]   "Néandertal Enterrait ses Morts", Musée de l'homme Paris, [*Online*]. Disponible en: https://www.museedelhomme.fr/fr/aller-plus-loin/dossiers/neandertal-enterrait-morts-4222.

[191]   Casado, M., "Forenses de Atapuerca tras las pistas del origen de los rituales funerarios", *El Correo de Burgos*, 29 may. 2022. [*Online*]. Disponible en: https://elcorreodeburgos.elmundo.es/articulo/burgos/forenses-pasado-pistas-origen-rituales-funerarios/20220528210853396941.html.

[192]   Casado, M., "Mtoto, el niño africano que despertó en Burgos", *El Correo de Burgos*, 6 may. 2021. [*Online*]. Disponible en: https://elcorreodeburgos.elmundo.es/articulo/burgos/mtoto-nino-africano-desperto-burgos/20210505194151377734.html.

[193]   Hume, D., *A Treatise of Human Nature*, London: A. D. Lindsay, 1911.

[194]   Darwin, C., *The Descent of Man*, New York: Modern Library, 1871.

[195]   Povinelli, D. J., *Folk Physics For Apes*, Oxford: Oxford University Press, 2003.

[196]   Povinelli, D. J., *Folks Physics for Apes*, New York: Oxford University Press, 2000.

[197]   Engelmann, J., "The Effects of Being Watched on Resource Acquisition in Chimpanzees and Human Children", *Animal Cognition*, vol. 19, pp. 147-51, 2016.

[198]   Meltzoff, B., "The Development of Gaze Following and Its Relation to Language", *Developmental science*, vol. 6, n.° 8, pp. 535-43, 2005.

[199]   Arsuaga, J. L., "La esencia humana", YouTube, [*Online*]. Disponible en: https://www.youtube.com/watch?v=3oyEeDJ7U7A.

[200]   Tomasello, M., *Becoming Human. A Theory of Ontogeny*, London: Harvard, 2021.

[201]   Arsuaga y Quian, "¿Qué nos hace humanos?", YouTube, 2022. [*Online*]. Disponible en: https://www.youtube.com/watch?v=Qm0Ts2fKA3M.

[202] Donaldson S. y Kymlicka, W., *Zoopolis A Political Theory of Animal Rights*, Oxford: Oxford University Press, 2014.

[203] Peterson, C., "25 years after returning to Yellowstone, wolves have helped stabilize the ecosystem", *National Geographic*, 10 jul. 2020.

[204] Sánchez, E., "Parques Nacionales autorizó la caza en solo un mes de 5.000 ciervos y jabalíes en Cabañeros", *El País*, 15 mar. 2022. [*Online*]. Disponible en: https://elpais.com/clima-y-medio-ambiente/2022-03-15/parques-nacionales-autorizo-la-caza-en-solo-un-mes-de-5000-ciervos-y-jabalies-en-cabaneros.html.

[205] Rothbard, M. N., *The Ethics of Liberty*, New York University Press, 1998.

[206] Cortina, A., *Las fronteras de la persona*, Hospitalet de Llobregat: Penguin Random House, 2009.

[207] Hart, H. L. A., "Are There Any Natural Rights", *The Philosophical Review*, vol. 64, n.° 2, pp. 175-191, 1955.

[208] Marks, J., *What it means to be 98% chimpanzee*, Berkeley: University of California Press, 2002.

[209] Ridley, M., "Matt Ridley blog", 6 jul. 2020. [*Online*]. Disponible en: https://www.rationaloptimist.com/blog/against-environmental-pessimism/.

[210] Fernández, M. A., "'El hombre no tiene naturaleza'. Un examen de la metafísica orteguiana", *Revista de filosofía*, vol. 45, n.° 1, pp. 69-85, 2020.

[211] Stenseth, N. C. "Mice, Rats, and People: The Bio-Economics of Agricultural Rodent Pests", *Frontiers in Ecology and the Environment*, vol 1 n.° 7, pp. 367-375, 2003.

[212] Brown, P. R., "Post-harvest damage to stored grain by rodents in village environments in Laos", *International Biodeterioration & Biodegradation 82* , pp. 104-109, 2013.

[213] Gebhardt, K., "A review and synthesis of bird and rodent damage estimates to select California Crops", *Crop Protection 30*, pp. 1109-1116, 2011.

[214] Guerri, J. F., "24 heures photo", *Le Figaro*, pp. https://www.lefigaro.fr/photos/24-heures-photo-du-22-fevrier-2021-20210222, 27 feb. 2021.

[215] Tovar, L., "La explotación de las abejas", 20 jun. 2015. [*Online*]. Disponible en: https://filosofiavegana.blogspot.com/2015/06/la-explotacion-de-las-abejas.html.

[216] FAO, "The Role, Impact and Welfare of Working Animals", Rome, 2011.

[217] PETA, "Animals are not Ours", [*Online*]. Disponible en: https://www.peta.org/issues/animals-in-entertainment/horse-drawn-carriages/.

[218] Schoenberg, N., "Chicago without horses: Activist wants to ban horse carriage operations, but owners deny animal cruelty", *Chicago Tribune*, 28 oct. 2019.

[219] LaPatilla, "Adiós a los paseos en carruaje por las calles de Roma", LaPatilla, 8 oct. 2018. [*Online*]. Disponible en: https://www.lapatilla.com/2018/10/08/adios-a-los-paseos-en-carruaje-por-las-calles-de-roma/?__cf_chl_managed_tk__=pmd_oAyPF.uMi6Eol5v7Nt96msjhMhgf6.pwyVUquMnz_mI-1632942520-0-gqNtZGzNAvu-jcnBszQi9.

[220] Sugy, P., "À Paris, les animalistes obtiennent des RTT pour les poneys... mais ne décolèrent pas", *Le Figaro*, 17 nov. 2021.

[221] Heparin Science, "Heparina. Una molécula que salva vidas", [*Online*]. Disponible en: https://www.heparinscience.com/heparina/.

[222] Ciencia explicada, "Poligelina". [*Online*]. Disponible en: https://cienciaexplicada.com/poligelina.html.

[223] Friendly, V., "Are Vaccines Vegan", [*Online*]. Disponible en: https://www.veganfriendly.org.uk/health-fitness/vaccines/.

[224] Buzz, T. V., "Egg-free flu-vaccine to save 50 million eggs a year", 10 oct. 2019. [*Online*]. Disponible en: https://www.totallyveganbuzz.com/news/egg-free-flu-vaccine-to-save-50-million-eggs-a-year/.

[225] Pascual, J., "Medicinas bestiales: tratamientos de origen animal (parte 1)", 30 ene. 2020. [*Online*]. Disponible en: https://naukas.com/2020/01/30/medicinas-bestiales-tratamientos-de-origen-animal-parte-1/.

[226]   UICN, "UICN", [*Online*]. Disponible en: https://www.iucn.org/es/node/19061.

[227]   Sous ses airs de peluche vivante, le vison d'Amérique est à bannir de Gironde. ActuBordeaux 31 juillet 2022. Disponible en: https://actu.fr/societe/sous-ses-airs-de-peluche-vivante-le-vison-d-amerique-est-a-bannir-de-gironde_52827470.html

[228]   Lahaine.org, "El Frente de Liberación Animal reivindica la liberación de 6500 visones y 19 gallinas", 14 abr. 2004. [*Online*]. Disponible en: https://www.lahaine.org/est_espanol.php/el-frente-de-liberacion-animal-1.

[229]   accionvegana.org, "Liberados 35.000 visones en Galicia", 11 jul. 2005. [*Online*]. Disponible en: http://barcelona.indymedia.org/newswire/display/191332.

[230]   Portela, R., "Especies invasoras (II): el visón americano", 4 abr. 2017. [*Online*]. Disponible en: https://cienciaybiologia.com/especies-invasoras-ii-vison-americano/.

[231]   Barrera, A., "Visón americano, la especie exótica invasora que arrasa con la fauna nativa", 9 feb. 2021. [*Online*]. Disponible en: https://www.bioguia.com/ambiente/vison-americano-la-especie-exotica-invasora-que-arrasa-con-la-fauna-nativa_89727506.html.

[232]   MAPA, "Estrategia de gestión, control y erradicación del visón americano (Neovison vison) en España", Ministerio de Agricultura, Alimentación y Medio Ambiente de España, Madrid, 2014.

[233]   Diario de Burgos, "CyL captura 8.000 visones americanos en las últimos 20 años", *Diario de Burgos*, 12 jun. 2021. [*Online*]. Disponible en: https://www.diariodeburgos.es/Noticia/ZFF54F767-AE49-6DBB-AA803765AAA60008/202106/CyL-captura-8000-visones-americanos-en-las-ultimos-20-anos.

[234]   Bayona, E.,"La costosa caza del visón americano, un portador de la COVID que invade ríos y lagunas", Eldiario.es, 28 mar. 2021. [*Online*]. Disponible en: https://www.eldiario.es/aragon/sociedad/costosa-caza-vison-americano-portador-covid-invade-rios-lagunas_1_7355373.html.

[235]   Natale, G., "Scholars and scientists in the history of the lymphatic system", *Journal of Anatomy*, vol. 3, n.° 231, pp. 417-429, 2017.

[236]   Dombrowski, D. A., *The philosophy of Vegetarianism*, Amherst: The University of Massachussetts Press, 1984.

[237]   Mayerson, H. S., "Three Centuries of Limphatic History – an Outline", *Lymphology*, vol. 2, pp. 143-150, 1969.

[238]   Franco, N. H., "Animal Experiments in Biomedical Research: A Historical Perspective", *Animals*, n.° 3, pp. 238-273, 2013.

[239]   Ecologistas en Acción, "Contra la experimentación animal", Ecologistas en Acción, 23 abr. 2012. [*Online*]. Disponible en: https://www.ecologistasenaccion.org/23060/contra-la-experimentacion-animal/. [Acceso 2 mar. 2021].

[240]   Barrecheguren, P., "Mayim Bialik y la experimentación animal", Naukas.com, 2 jun. 2017. [*Online*]. Disponible en: https://naukas.com/2017/06/02/mayim-bialik-la-experimentacion-animal/. [Acceso 2 mar. 2021].

[241]   CNIO, "III Jornada CNIO-Fundación Sabadell en filosofía y ciencia", YouTube, 23 nov. 2021. [*Online*]. Disponible en: https://www.youtube.com/watch?v=sVsHBj-eY91E.

[242]   "Scientific Arguments Against Animal Experiments", Doctors Against Animals Experiments, [*Online*]. Disponible en: https://aerzte-gegen-tierversuche.de/en/. [Acceso 2 mar. 2021].

[243]   HSUS, "YouTube", Human Society of The United States, [*Online*]. Disponible en: https://www.youtube.com/watch?v=BQn3NaJgYnI. [Acceso 2 mar. 2021].

[244]   "What animals are used in coronavirus research", European Animal Research Association, 16 abr. 2020. [*Online*]. Disponible en: https://www.eara.eu/post/what-animals-are-used-in-coronavirus-research?lang=es. [Acceso 2 mar. 2021].

[245]   Álvarez, C., "Sin experimentación animal, no tendríamos ahora vacunas contra la covid", *El País*, 14 abr. 2021. [*Online*]. Disponible en: https://elpais.com/clima-y-medio-ambiente/2021-04-14/sin-experimentacion-animal-no-tendriamos-ahora-vacunas-contra-la-covid.html.

[246]   Kordower, J. H., "Animal Rights Terrorists: What Every Neuroscientist Should Know", *Journal of Neuroscience*, vol. 37, n.° 29, p. 11419-11420, 2009.

[247]   Abbott, A., "Animal-rights activists wreak havoc in Milan laboratory", *Nature News*, 22 abr. 2013.

[248]   "CAMPUS LIFE: Michigan State; Animal Rights Raiders Destroy Years of Work", *The New York Times*, p. 51, 8 mar. 1992.

[249]   APA, "APA Condemns Vandalism at University of Iowa Lab Facilit", *American Psycological Association*, nov. 2004.

[250]   AMP, "The Critical Role of Animals in Developing COVID-19 Treatments and Vaccines", Americans for Medical Progress, 2021. [*Online*]. Disponible en: https://www.amprogress.org/covid-19-resources/covid19animalresearch/. [Acceso 2 mar. 2021].

[251]   NABR, "The Importance of Animal Research", NABR, 2020. [*Online*]. Disponible en: https://www.nabr.org/biomedical-research/importance-biomedical-research#. [Acceso 8 mar. 2021].

[252]   Harvard, "Animal Studies", Harvard, 2021. [*Online*]. Disponible en: https://vpr.harvard.edu/pages/animal-studies. [Acceso 8 mar. 2021].

[253]   Stanford University, "Why Animal Research", Animal Research at Stanford, [*Online*]. Disponible en: https://med.stanford.edu/animalresearch/why-animal-research.html. [Acceso 8 Mar 2021].

[254]   M. instituciones, "French transparency Charter on the use of animals", 22 feb. 2021. [*Online*]. Disponible en: https://www.recherche-animale.org/sites/default/files/french_transparency_charter_animals_for_science_-_22feb21-_eng.pdf. [Acceso 8 mar. 2021].

[255]   T. B. Declaration, "Basel Declaration", 2010. [*Online*]. Disponible en: https://www.basel-declaration.org/basel-declaration/. [Acceso 8 mar. 2021].

[256]   Utilisation d'animaux à des fins scientifiques dans les établissements français – Enquête statistique 2021 – Direction générale de la recherche et de l'innovation. Ministère de l'enseignement supérieure et de la recherche. Disponible en: https://www.enseignementsup-recherche.gouv.fr/sites/default/files/2023-02/enqu-te-2021-utilisation-des-animaux-des-fins-scientifiques-26480.pdf

[257]   Unión Europea, "Diario Oficial de la Unión Europea", 20 Oct 2010. [*Online*]. Disponible en: https://eur-lex.europa.eu/legal-content/ES/TXT/PDF/?uri=CELEX-:32010L0063&from=EN. [Acceso 8 mar. 2021].

[258]   Pro-Test, "Pro-Test", Pro-Test Standing Up for Science, 2006. [*Online*]. Disponible en: http://www.pro-test.org.uk/facts.php?lt=b. [Acceso 8 mar. 2021].

[259]   Botting, J., "The History of Thalidomide. Drug News Perspective", *Drug News Perspect.*, vol. 15, n.° 9, pp. 604-611, 2002.

[260]   NY Times, "19,000 Animals Killed in Automotive Crash Tests", *The New York Times*, p. 26, 28 sep. 1991.

[261]   C. Europea, "Informe de la Comisión al Parlamento Europeo y al Consejo sobre el desarrollo, la validación y la aceptación legal de métodos alternativos a la experimentación con animales en el ámbito de los cosméticos", 15 oct. 2019.

[262]   Abbot, A., "The lowdown on animal testing for cosmetics", *Nature*, https://www.nature.com/news/2009/090311/full/news.2009.147.html, 11 mar. 2009.

[263]   Diario Veterinario, "Cómo la veterinaria contribuye al avance de la medicina humana", 3 March 2021. [*Online*]. Disponible en: https://www.diarioveterinario.com/t/2695823/como-veterinaria-contribuye-avance-medicina-humana.

[264]   Gircor, "La retraite des animaux de laboratoire", abr. 2018. [*Online*]. Disponible en: https://www.recherche-animale.org/sites/default/files/brochure_gircor_bat.pdf.

[265]   Whiterabbit.org, "Whiterabbit.org", [*Online*]. Disponible en: https://www.white-rabbit.org/.

[266]   SIMV, "Recours à l'animal au sein des laboratoires pharmaceutiques vétérinaires", SIMV, 2020. [*Online*]. Disponible en: https://intranet.simv.org/sites/default/files/u1611/contexte_du_recours_aux_animaux_a_des_fins_scientifiques_ou_reglementaires_version_finale_280721.pdf.

[267]   Finances Online, "Number of Dogs in the US 2021/2022: Statistics, Demographics, and Trends", Finance Online, [Online]. Disponible en: https://financesOnline.com/number-of-dogs-in-the-us/.

[268]   AVMA, "U.S. pet ownership statistics", AMVA, [Online]. Disponible en: https://www.avma.org/resources-tools/reports-statistics/us-pet-ownership-statistics.

[269]   "Combien de chats en france – population de chats en france : tout savoir", J'aime trop chat, 30 jun. 2020. [Online]. Disponible en: https://www.jaimetropchat.fr/tout-savoir-population-chats-france/.

[270]   Chien.com, 2 feb. 2020. [Online]. Disponible en: https://www.chien.com/le-chien-50/les-10-pays-d-europe-qui-comptent-le-plus-de-chiens-la-france-18491-4_5.php.

[271]   Statista, "Número de gatos como animales de compañía en España de 2010 a 2020", Statista, 26 ago. 2021. [Online]. Disponible en: https://es.statista.com/esta-disticas/592973/numero-de-gatos-en-espana/.

[272]   SrPerro, "Los perros en España, algunas cifras: casi 7 millones de canes en 2019", SrPerro, 2019. [Online]. Disponible en: https://www.srperro.com/consejos/curiosi-dades/los-perros-en-espana-algunas-cifras/.

[273]   Durán, V., "Mascotas, un negocio que mueve 36.500 millones de euros al año en la Unión Europea", Expansión, 9 oct. 2018. [Online]. Disponible en: https://www.ex-pansion.com/directivos/estilo-vida/2018/10/06/5bb7603522601de9538b45ef.html.

[274]   Francione G. y Charlton, A. E., "The case against pets", AEON, 8 sep. 2016. [On-line]. Disponible en: https://aeon.co/essays/why-keeping-a-pet-is-fundamentally-un-ethical.

[275]   Coppinger, R.,What Is A Dog, Chicago: The University of Chicago Press, 2016.

[276]   Hendriks, W., "The omnivorous dog dogma and carnivorous cat connection", in ESVCN - European Society of Veterinary and Comparitive Nutrition, Utrech, 2014.

[277]   Heinze, C. R., "Vegan Dogs – A healthy lifestyle or going against nature?", Clinical Nutrition Service, pp. https://vetnutrition.tufts.edu/2016/07/vegan-dogs-a-healthy-lifestyle-or-going-against-nature/, 21 jul. 2016.

[278]   Grinber, E., "Vegan diet for dogs: A question of thriving vs. surviving", CNN, 10 mar. 2011. [Online]. Disponible en: http://edition.cnn.com/2011/LIVING/03/10/vegan.dog.diet/.

[279]   British Veterinary Association, "Should dogs and cats be fed a vegan diet? BVA issues statement in response to media flurry", British Veterinary Association, 22 oct. 2021. [Online]. Disponible en: https://www.bva.co.uk/news-and-blog/news-article/should-dogs-and-cats-be-fed-a-vegan-diet-bva-issues-statement-in-response-to-media-flurry/.

[280]   Lowe, R., "Vegan diets are healthier and safer for dogs – or are they?", VetHelp-Direct, 15 abr. 2022. [Online]. Disponible en: https://vethelpdirect.com/vet-blog/2022/04/15/vegan-diets-are-healthier-and-safer-for-dogs-or-are-they/.

[281]   Hawn, R., "Should Your Pet Go on a Vegetarian Diet?", WebMD, 19 may. 2011. [On-line]. Disponible en: https://pets.webmd.com/features/vegetarian-diet-dogs-cats#1.

[282]   Clarkson, N., "Horses as meat eating killers", The Long Riders Guild Academic Foundation, [Online]. Disponible en: http://www.lrgaf.org/Deadly%20Equines%20-%20Review%20in%20Horse%20Connection.pdf.

[283]   Khully, P., "One Vet's Advice: Don't Force Your Pet to Be Vegan", VetStreet, pp. http://www.vetstreet.com/our-pet-experts/one-vets-advice-dont-force-your-pet-to-be-vegan, 15 jul. 2014.

[284]   Huston, L., "Vegan Diets for Cats", PetMD, pp. https://www.petmd.com/blogs/the-dailyvet/lorieahuston/2014/june/vegan-diets-cats-31822, 17 jun. 2014.

[285]   Becker, K. S., "Why cats can't be vegetarian", Animal Wellness, pp. https://animal-wellnessmagazine.com/cats-cant-vegetarian/, 27 dic. 2017.

[286]   Drake, J., "Vegan Cat Food for Carnivorous Felines?", Hills, pp. https://www.hills-pet.com/cat-care/nutrition-feeding/vegan-cat-food-concerns, 2 feb. 2016.

[287]   Cecchetti, M. *et al.*, "Contributions of wild and provisioned foods to the diets of domestic cats that depredate wild animals", *Ecosphere*, vol. 12, n.º 9, p. e03737, 2021.

[288]   Trouwborst, A., McCormack, P. C., y Camacho, E. M., "Domestic cats and their impacts on biodiversity: A blind spot in the application of nature conservation law", *People and Nature*, vol. 2, n.º 1, pp. 235-250, 2020.

[289]   Loss, S. R. *et al.*, "The impact of free-ranging domestic cats on Wildlife in the United States", *Nature communications*, 2012.

[290]   PACMA, "Método CER: regularemos las colonias felinas de manera ética", PACMA, 16 may. 2019. [*Online*]. Disponible en: https://elecciones.pacma.es/elecciones-2019/diario/metodo-cer-regularemos-las-colonias-felinas-de-manera-etica/.

[291]   Pavés, V., "Los gatos ponen en jaque la supervivencia del lagarto gigante de Tenerife", *El día. La opinión de Tenerife*, 16 mar. 2022. [*Online*]. Disponible en: https://www.eldia.es/sociedad/2022/03/16/gatos-ponen-jaque-supervivencia-lagarto-63910704.html.

[292]   Padilla, Á., "La lucha animalista en España: presente y porvenir XIII", El periodic.com, 13 jul. 2021. [*Online*]. Disponible en: https://www.elperiodic.com/opinion/yo-animal/lucha-animalista-espana-presente-porvenir-xiii_8028.

[293]   Masters, B., "Wild Horses: The Consequences of Doing Nothing", *National Geographic*, 7 feb. 2017. [*Online*]. Disponible en: https://www.nationalgeographic.com/adventure/article/wild-horses-part-two.

[294]   RUBINOFF, D., y LEPCZYK, C.,"Wild Horses Are Terrible for the West", Slate, 14 dic. 2015. [*Online*]. Disponible en: https://slate.com/technology/2015/12/wild-feral-horses-are-bad-for-the-environment-in-the-west.html.

[295]   Gerber, P. J. *et al.*, "Tackling climate change through livestock – A global assessment of emissions and mitigation", FAO, Roma, 2013.

[296]   Eurostat, "Statistics Explained (https://ec.europa.eu/eurostat/statistics-explained/index.php?title=File:Figure_1_Contribution_of_agriculture_to_total_GHG_emissions_(%25),_EU-28,_2015.png)", Eurostat, 2019.

[297]   United States Environmental Protection Agency, "Greenhouse Gas Emissions", EPA, 2019.

[298]   FAO, "Tackling Climate Change through Livestock", FAO, Rome, 2013.

[299]   Mitloehner, F., "Using Global Emission Statistics is Distracting Us From Climate Change Solutions", Clear Center UC Davis, 2020.

[300]   Our World in Data, "Methane Emissions", Our World in Data, 2016. [*Online*]. Disponible en: https://ourworldindata.org/grapher/methane-emissions?tab=chart.

[301]   Felisa A. Smith *et al.*, "Exploring the influence of ancient and historic megaherbivore extirpations on the global Methane Budget", *PNAS*, pp. 874-879, 2016.

[302]   Hristov, A., "Historic, pre-European settlement, and present-day contribution of Wild Ruminants to Enteric Emissions in the United States", *Journal of Animal Science*, pp. 1371-1375, 2012.

[303]   P. Manzano and S. White, "Greenhouse gas emissions from pastoral livestock systems versus alternative landmanagement scenarios", [*Online*]. Disponible en: https://helda.helsinki.fi//bitstream/handle/10138/326549/Intensifying_pastoralism_AAM.pdf?sequence=1.

[304]   White, R. y Hall, M., "Nutritional and greenhouse gas impacts of removing animals from US agriculture", *Proceedings of the National Academy of Sciences*, 2017.

[305]   "L'empreinte carbone des français, un sujet tabou ?", *Ravijen blog*, Disponible en: https://ravijen.fr/?p=440, 2018.

[306]   Lomborg, B., "Where's the beef? Ask green campaigners", *Shine beyond a single story*, 30 nov. 2018.

[307]   Kanemoto, K. *et al.*, "Meat Consumption Does Not Explain Differences in Household Food Carbon Footprints in Japan", *One Earth*, pp. 464-471, 2019.

[308]   https://foodandagricultureorganization.shinyapps.io/GLEAMV3_Public/

[309] Lynch, J. *et al.*, "Demonstrating GWP*: a means of reporting warming-equivalent emissions that captures the contrasting impacts of short- and long-lived climate pollutants", *Environ. Res. Lett.*, 2020.

[310] IPCC, "AR6 Climate Change 2021: The Physical Science Basis", IPCC, 2021.

[311] Skeptical Science, "Does breathing contribute to CO2 buildup in the atmosphere?", Skeptical Science, 13 Sep 2018. [*Online*]. Disponible en: https://skepticalscience.com/breathing-co2-carbon-dioxide.htm.

[312] Allen, M., "Conversations That Matter: Are cows getting a bad GHG Rap?", YouTube. [*Online*]. Disponible en: https://www.youtube.com/watch?v=brOuHKr0snM.

[313] Rowntree J. E. *et al.*, "Ecosystem Impacts and Productive Capacity of a Multi-Species Pastured Livestock System", *Frontiers in Sustainable Food Systems*, p. 232, 2020.

[314] Cymru, H. C., "The Welsh Way: Towards Global Leadership in Sustainable Lamb and Beef Production", *Meat Promotion Wales*, pp. 25-26, 2020.

[315] Carrasco, A. F., "Así ha bajado la contaminación durante el estado de alarma por el coronavirus", Greenpeace, 19 mar. 2020. [*Online*]. Disponible en: https://es.greenpeace.org/es/noticias/asi-ha-bajado-la-contaminacion-durante-el-estado-de-alarma-por-el-coronavirus/.

[316] Greenpeace, "Open letter on improving air quality to save lives after lockdown", Greenpeace, 11 may. 2020. [*Online*]. Disponible en: https://www.greenpeace.org.uk/resources/open-letter-on-improving-air-quality-to-save-lives-after-lockdown/.

[317] Sonno, T. *et al.*, "Pollution reductions during lockdowns can teach us how to build back better a sustainable economy", *Vox EU CEPR Research-based policy analysis and commentary from leading economists*, 21 jun. 2021.

[318] Frankowska, A. *et al.*, "Environmental impacts of vegetables consumption in the UK", *Science of The Total Environment*, pp. 80-105, 2019.

[319] Our World In Data, "CO2 footprint", Our World In Data, [*Online*]. Disponible en: https://ourworldindata.org/food-choice-vs-eating-local.

[320] Drewnowski, A., "Energy and nutrient density of foods in relation to their carbon footprint", *The American Journal of Clinical Nutrition*, vol. 101, n.º 1, pp. 184-191, 2015.

[321] Statista, "Share of food wasted globally as of 2017, by food category", Statista, 2017. [*Online*]. Disponible en: https://www.statista.com/statistics/519611/percentage-of-wasted-food-by-category-global/.

[322] MAPA, "El desperdicio alimentario en los hogares españoles aumentó un 8,9% en 2018", MAPA, 19 jun. 2019. [*Online*]. Disponible en: https://www.mapa.gob.es/es/prensa/190619desperdicioalimentariov2_tcm30-510666.pdf.

[323] González-Recio, Ó., "Esta es la huella ambiental de la comida que tiramos a la basura", The Conversation, 22 dic. 2019. [*Online*]. Disponible en: https://theconversation.com/esta-es-la-huella-ambiental-de-la-comida-que-tiramos-a-la-basura-128797.

[324] Conrad, Z. *et al.*, "Relationship between food waste, diet quality, and environmental sustainability", *PLOS ONE*, p. 13 (4), 2018.

[325] Skeptical Science, 19 mar. 2020. [*Online*]. Disponible en: https://skepticalscience.com/vegan_reduce_greenhouse_gas_emissions.html.

[326] Heller, M. C. *et al.*, "Toward a Life Cycle-Based, Diet-level Framework for Food Environmental Impact and Nutritional Quality Assessment: A Critical", *Environmental Science Technology*, pp. 12632-12647, 2013.

[327] Carlsson-Kanyama, A., y González, A., "Potential contributions of food consumption patterns to climate change", *The American Journal of Clinical Nutrition*, pp. 1704S-1709S, 2009.

[328] FAO, "The state of the world's land and water resources for food and water resources for food and agriculture (SOLAW) -Managing systems at risk", Rome, 2011.

[329] FAO, "Statistical Yearbook", Rome, 2020.

[330] Mitloehner, F., "How Much Land Is Used for Livestock", YouTube, [*Online*]. Disponible en: https://www.youtube.com/watch?v=rvIGxFvBR0c&t=113s.

[331]   Ranum, P. et al., "Global maize production, utilization, and consumption", *Annals of the New York Academy Of Sciences*, vol. 1312, pp. 105-112, 2014.

[332]   Mottet, A., "Livestock: On our plates or eating at our table?. A niew analysis of the feed/food debate", *Global Food Security*, 2017.

[333]   Meindertsma, C., *Pig 05049*, Flocks, 2007.

[334]   Song, XP., Hansen, M.C., Stehman, S.V. et al. Global land change from 1982 to 2016. Nature 560, 639–643 (2018). https://doi.org/10.1038/s41586-018-0411-9.

[335]   State of Europe's Forests 2020. https://foresteurope.org/wp-content/uploads/2016/08/SoEF_2020.pdf.

[336]   https://gfcommodities.com/blog/commercial-uses-for-recycled-cooking-oil/.

[337]   https://www.darpro-solutions.com/media/blog/second-life-for-used-cooking-oil-and-animal-fats.

[338]   Service public Fédéral de la Santé publique, de la Sécurité de la Chaîne alimentaire et de l'Environnement. Alimentation végétarienne. Abril. 2021. https://www.health.belgium.be/sites/default/files/uploads/fields/fpshealth_theme_file/210409_css-9445_alimentation_vegetarienne_vweb_0.pdf

[339]   Fewtrell, Mary et al. Complementary Feeding: A Position Paper by the European Society for Paediatric Gastroenterology, Hepatology, and Nutrition (ESPGHAN) Committee on Nutrition. Journal of Pediatric Gastroenterology and Nutrition. 2017. 119-132. 64 (1)

[340]   Richter, M. et al., "Vegan Diet. Position of the German Nutrition Society", Ernahrungs Umschau, vol. 63, n.° 4, pp. 92-102, 2016.

[341]   Kersting, M. et al., "Vegetarian Diets in Children? - An Assessment from Pediatrics and Nutrition Science", Deutsche Medizinische Wochenschrift, vol. 143, n.° 4, pp. 279-286, 2018.

[342]   Khan, S., "Belgian Doctors Say Vegan Diet is Not Healthy for Kids", Science Times, 21 may. 2019. [*Online*]. Disponible en: https://www.sciencetimes.com/articles/21989/20190521/belgian-doctors-say-vegan-diet-is-not-healthy-for-kids.htm.

[343]   Federal Commission for Nutrition. (FCN), "Vegan diets: review of nutritional benefits and risks. Expert report of the FCN", FCN, Berna, 2018.

[344]   Redecilla, S. et al., "Recomendaciones del Comité de Nutrición y Lactancia Materna de la Asociación Española de Pediatría sobre las dietas vegetarianas", *Anales de Pediatría*, vol. 92, n.° 5, pp. 306.e1-306.e6, 2020.

[345]   Merritt, R. J. et al., "Plant-based Milks, Journal of Pediatric Gastroenterology and Nutrition", *Journal of Pediatric Gastroenterology and Nutrition*, vol. 71, n.° 2, pp. 276-281, 2020.

[346]   Lund, A. M., "Questions about a vegan diet should be included in differential diagnostics of neurologically abnormal infants with failure to thrive", *Acta Paediatrica*, vol. 108, n.° 8, pp. 1377-1379, 2019.

[347]   Lemale J. et al., "Vegan diet in children and adolescents. Recommendations from the French-speaking Pediatric Hepatology, Gastroenterology and Nutrition Group (GFHGNP)", *Archives de Pediatrie*, vol. 26, n.° 7, pp. 442-450, 2019.

[348]   FSAI 1-5 Year-Olds, Food Safety Ireland, 22 jun. 2020. [*Online*]. Disponible en: https://www.fsai.ie/news_centre/press_releases/healthy_eating_1-5year-olds_22062020.html.

[349]   Mauro G. et al., "Position paper SIPPS-FIMP-SIMP diete vegetariane in gravidanza ed età evolutiva", SIPPS FIMP SIMP, 2017.

[350]   Melina, V. et al., "Position of the Academy of Nutrition and Dietetics: Vegetarian Diets", *Journal of the Academy of Nutrition and Dietetics*, vol. 116, n.° 12, pp. 1970-1980, 2016.

[351]   Hayes, D., "Feeding Vegetarian and Vegan Infants and Toddlers", 23 Oct 2019. [*Online*]. Disponible en: https://www.eatright.org/food/nutrition/vegetarian-and-special-diets/feeding-vegetarian-and-vegan-infants-and-toddlers.

[352] India.com, "Anaemia Cases on Rise Across India: Check Cause, Symptoms, Treatment HERE", India.com, 28 may. 2022. [*Online*]. Disponible en: https://www.india.com/health/anaemia-cases-on-rise-across-india-check-cause-symptoms-treatment-here-5417327/.

[353] Baños, J. J., "Carnívoros, a las catacumbas", *La Vanguardia*, 23 nov. 2021.

[354] López, A., "India enfrenta una invasión de vacas abandonadas que mueren de hambre en las calles", *National Geographic Español*, 7 feb. 2021.

[355] FAO, "The State of Food Security and Nutrition in the World 2020", FAO, Rome, 2020.

[356] Beal, T. y Ortenzi, F., "Priority micronutrient density in foods", *Research Square*, p. Pre print version, 2021.

[357] "Micronutrient Density of Foods for Complementary Feeding of Young Children (6-23 months) in South and South East Asia", *Frontiers in Nutrition*, vol. 8, 2021.

[358] Beal, T. y Ortenzi, F., "Priority Micronutrient Density in Foods", *Research Square*, 2021.

[359] Tarnowski, C., "Preventing and treating an iron deficiency", mysportscience.com, [*Online*]. Disponible en: https://www.mysportscience.com/post/preventing-and-treating-iron-deficiency.

[360] Roohani, N. *et al.*, "Zinc and its importance for human health: An integrative review", *Journal of research in medical sciences : the official journal of Isfahan University of Medical Sciences*, vol. 18, n.° 2, pp. 144-157, 2013.

[361] Tang, G., "Bioconversion of dietary provitamin A carotenoids to vitamin A in humans", *American Journal of Clinic Nutrition*, vol. 91, p. 1468S-73S, 2010.

[362] Iguacel, I. *et al.*, "Veganism, vegetarianism, bone mineral density, and fracture risk: a systematic review and meta-analysis", *Nutrition Reviews*, vol. 77, n.° 1, pp. 1-18, 2019.

[363] Grasgruber, P. *et al.*, "Major correlates of male height: A study of 105 countries", *Economics and Human Biology*, vol. 21, pp. 172-195, 2016.

[364] Headey, D., y Palloni, G., "Stunting and Wasting Among Indian Preschoolers have Moderate but Significant Associations with the Vegetarian Status of their Mothers", *The Journal of Nutrition*, vol. 150, n.° 6, pp. 1579-1589.

[365] Awidi, M. *et al.*, "Contributing factors to iron deficiency anemia in women in Jordan: A single-center crosssectional study", *PLOS ONE*, vol. 13, n.° 11, p. e0205868, 2018.

[366] Sun, H. y Weaver, C., "Decreased Iron Intake Parallels Rising Iron Deficiency Anemia and Related Mortality Rates in the US Population", *The Journal of Nutrition*, vol. 151, n.° 7, pp. 1947-1955, 2021.

[367] Pawlak, R. *et al*, "Iron Status of Vegetarian Adults: A Review of Literature", *Am J Lifestyle Med*, vol. 12, n.° 6, pp. 486-498, 2016.

[368] Pawlak, R. *et al.*, "Iron Status of Vegetarian Adults: A Review of Literature", *American Journal of Lifestyle Medicine*, vol. 12 , n.°. 6, pp. 486-498, 2018.

[369] Redacción, "Advierten de que aumentan los casos de anemia en mujeres", *La Voz de Galicia*, 21 abr. 2022. [*Online*]. Disponible en: https://www.lavozdegalicia.es/noticia/sociedad/2022/04/21/aumentan-casos-anemia-mujeres-vegetarianas/00031650557210698334779.htm.

[370] Valle, S., "La dieta vegetariana es la causa, cada vez más frecuente, de anemia ferropénica en mujeres", *Diario Médico*, 22 abr. 2022. [*Online*]. Disponible en: https://www.diariomedico.com/medicina/ginecologia/profesion/la-dieta-vegetariana-es-la-causa-cada-vez-mas-frecuente-de-anemia-ferropenica-en-mujeres.html.

[371] Dobersek, U. *et al.*, "Meat and mental health: a systematic review of meat abstention and depression, anxiety, and related phenomena", *Critical Reviews in Food Science and Nutrition*, vol. 61, n.° 4, pp. 622-635, 2021.

[372] Aubertin-Leheudre, M. y Adlercreutz, H., "Relationship between animal protein intake and muscle mass index in healthy women", *Br J Nutr.*, vol. 102, n.° 12, pp. 1803-10, 2009.

[373] Domić, J. et al., "Perspective: Vegan Diets for Older Adults? A Perspective On the Potential Impact On Muscle Mass and Strength", *Adv Nutr*, vol. 13, n.° 3, pp. 712-725, 2022.

[374] Pascual, J., "A vueltas con la Vitamina B$_{12}$", Naukas.com, 2 sep. 2020. [*Online*]. Disponible en: https://naukas.com/2020/09/02/a-vueltas-con-la-vitamina-b12/.

[375] Fang, H. et al., "Microbial production of vitamin B$_{12}$: a review and future perspectives", *Microb Cell Fact*, vol. 16, n.° 15, 2017.

[376] Heinrich Böll Stiftung, "Meat Atlas 2021", Heinrich Böll Stiftung, Friends of the Earth, Bund für Umwelt und Naturschutz, 2021.

[377] Dam, A., "Right to food: The politics of vegetarianism in India", The Telegraph *Online*, 23 nov. 2019. [*Online*]. Disponible en: https://www.telegraphindia.com/health/right-to-food-the-politics-of-vegetarianism-in-india/cid/1721235.

[378] Karpagam, S. et al., "India Shows Why The Global Shift To Plant-Based Diets Is Dangerous", Ozy, 4 Dec 2019. [*Online*]. Disponible en: https://www.ozy.com/around-the-world/india-shows-why-the-global-shift-to-plant-based-diets-is-dangerous/250958/.

[379] Nordhaus, T., "In Sri Lanka, Organic Farming Went Catastrophically Wrong", *Foreing Policy*, 5 mar. 2022.

[380] Mugerwa, E. N., "Criticism of animal farming in the west risks health of world's poorest", *The Guardian*, 10 sep. 2021.

[381] EAT, "The EAT-Lancet Commission on Food, Planet, Health", EAT, [*Online*]. Disponible en: https://eatforum.org/eat-lancet-commission/.

[382] Karpagam, S. et al., "India Shows Why The Global Shift To Plant-Based Diets Is Dangerous", OZY, 4 Dec 2019. [*Online*]. Disponible en: https://www.ozy.com/around-the-world/india-shows-why-the-global-shift-to-plant-based-diets-is-dangerous/250958/.

[383] Wikipedia, "Bushmeat", Wikipedia, [*Online*]. Disponible en: https://en.wikipedia.org/wiki/Bushmeat.

[384] Sainz, L., "Dietas de carne y lácteos aumentan 12% el riesgo de cáncer de mama: estudio", Veganizatuvida.com, 15 Junio 2021. [*Online*]. Disponible en: https://veganizatuvida.com/dietas-de-carne-y-lacteos-aumentan-12-el-riesgo-de-cancer-de-mama-estudio.

[385] IARC, "Agents Classified by the IARC Monographs, volumes 1-129", IARC, 22 jul. 2021. [*Online*]. Disponible en: https://monographs.iarc.who.int/agents-classified-by-the-iarc/.

[386] Mulet J. M., "Carnes roja, cáncer y otros mitos alimentarios", *El escéptico*, pp. 30-31, 2015.

[387] Wikipedia, "List of IARC Group 2A Agents - Probably carcinogenic to humans", Wikipedia, [*Online*]. Disponible en: https://en.wikipedia.org/wiki/List_of_IARC_Group_2A_Agents_-_Probably_carcinogenic_to_humans.

[388] IARC, "Press Release 240", WHO, 26 oct. 2015. [*Online*]. Disponible en: https://www.iarc.who.int/wp-content/uploads/2018/07/pr240_E.pdf.

[389] Guyatt, G., "Think beef", feb. 2018. [*Online*]. Disponible en: https://thinkbeef.ca/wp-content/uploads/2018/03/Mistaken-Advice-on-Red-Meat-and-Cancer_May9.pdf.

[390] Guyatt, G., "A False Alarm on Red Meat and Cancer", *Financial Times*, 24 nov. 2015.

[391] Gideon M-K, "Bacon is not the enemy", Gidmk, 18 abr. 2019. [*Online*]. Disponible en: https://gidmk.medium.com/bacon-is-not-the-enemy-bd861c2adac9.

[392] Aaron E. Carroll, et al., "Meat Consumption and Health: Food for Thought", *Annals of Internal Medecine*, 2019.

[393] Rubin, R., "Backlash Over Meat Dietary Recommendations Raises Questions", *Journal of American Medical Association*, pp. E1-E4, 2020.

[394] INE, "Esperanza de Vida", Instituto Nacional de Estadística de España, 2019. [*Online*]. Disponible en: https://www.ine.es/ss/Satellite?c=INESeccion_C&cid=1259926380048&p=1254735110672&pagename=ProductosYServicios%2FPYSLayout.

[395] Wikipedia, "Trans fat", Wikipedia, [*Online*]. Disponible en: https://en.wikipedia.org/wiki/Trans_fat.

[396] Wikipedia, "Trans fat regulation", Wikipedia, [*Online*]. Disponible en: https://en-.wikipedia.org/wiki/Trans_fat_regulation.

[397] Ku S. K. *et al.*, "The harmful effects of consumption of repeatedly heated edible oils: a short review", *Clin. Ter.*, vol. 165, n.° 4, pp. 217-221, 2014.

[398] Ng, Chun-Yi *et al.*, "Heated vegetable oils and cardiovascular disease risk factors", *Vascul Pharmacol* , vol. 61, n.° 1, pp. 1-9, 2014.

[399] Appleby, P. *et al.*, "Mortality in vegetarians and comparable nonvegetarians in the United Kingdom", *The American Journal of Clinical Nutrition*, vol. 103, n.° 1, pp. 218-230, 2016.

[400] Timothy J. Key *et al.*,"Cancer incidence in vegetarians: results from the European Prospective Investigation into Cancer and Nutrition (EPIC-Oxford)", *The American Journal of Clinic,* vol. 89, n.° 5, pp. 1620S-1626S, 2009.

[401] Dombrowski, D. A., *The Philosophy Of Vegetarianism*, Amherst: The University of Massachusetts Press, 1984.

[402] Erlenbush, R., "Why do Catholics Abstain from Meat?", The New Theological Movement, 21 Mar 2012. [*Online*]. Disponible en: https://newtheologicalmovement.blogspot.com/2012/03/why-do-catholics-abstain-from-meat.html.

[403] Mazokopakis E. E., "Why is Meat Excluded from the Orthodox Christian Diet during Fasting? A Religious and Medical Approach", *Maedica*, vol. 13, n.° 4, pp. 282-285, 2018.

[404] Markel, H., *The Kelloggs*, New York: Vintage Books, 2017.

[405] Roy, P., "Meat-Eating, Masculinity, and Renunciation in India: A Gandhian Grammar of Diet", *Gender & History* , vol. 14, n.° 1, pp. 62-91, 2002.

[406] T. E. S. o. B. Buddhism, "False beliefs. Book two", The Eastern School of Broad Buddhism, 2005. [*Online*]. Disponible en: http://www.meherbabadnyana.net/life_eternal/Book_Two/2_False_Beliefs.htm#03.

[407] Today, H., "Vegetarianism and Meat-Eating in 8 Religions", *Hinduism Today*, 1 Apr 2007. [*Online*]. Disponible en: https://www.hinduismtoday.com/magazine/april-may-june-2007/2007-04-vegetarianism-and-meat-eating-in-8-religions/.

[408] Redacción, "Menus sans viande à Lyon : la mairie écologiste annonce le retour de la viande dans les cantines scolaires", *Le Figaro*, 14 abr. 2021. [*Online*]. Disponible en: https://www.lefigaro.fr/politique/menus-sans-viande-a-lyon-la-mairie-ecologiste-annonce-le-retour-de-la-viande-dans-les-cantines-scolaires-20210414.

[409] Rodgers, D., "Feeding the World a Healthy and Sustainable Diet? How EAT Lancet Gets it Wrong", YouTube, [*Online*]. Disponible en: https://www.youtube.com/watch?v=kNDmp6C1IAM.

[410] The New York Post, "Plant-Powered Meals", *The New York Post*, 3 feb. 2022. [*Online*]. Disponible en: https://nypost.com/2022/02/03/nyc-schools-to-serve-vegan-only-meals-on-fridays/.

[411] Eater New York, "'Vegan' Mayor Eric Adams Under Fire for Repeatedly Ordering Fish at NYC Restaurants", *Eater New York*, 28 Feb 2022. [*Online*]. Disponible en: https://ny.eater.com/2022/2/8/22921907/vegan-nyc-mayor-eric-adams-under-fire-eats-fish.

[412] Rowe, M., "Portland elementary schools dish up daily hot vegan option", *Food Management*, 24 Mar 2022. [*Online*]. Disponible en: https://www.food-management.com/k-12-schools/portland-elementary-schools-dish-daily-hot-vegan-option.

[413] "Netherlands: Concept of a Meat Tax Under Discussion in the Netherlands", USDA Foreign Agricultural Service, 29 jun. 2022. [*Online*]. Disponible en: https://www.fas.usda.gov/data/netherlands-concept-meat-tax-under-discussion-netherlands.

[414] "Meat Is The New Tobacco", *Huffpost*, 6 Dec 2017. [*Online*]. Disponible en: https://www.huffpost.com/entry/animal-products-cancer_b_1316222.